Speaking of Women's Health

D0062686

The Book

This beautiful song was written by Jana Stanfield and Jimmy Scott and is often sung by Jana when she presents at our Speaking of Women's Health conferences. Jana dedicated this song to the women across America, who hold in their hearts the spirit of Speaking of Women's Health!

If I Were Brave?

What would I do if I knew that I could not fail?
If I believed would the wind always fill up my sail?
How far would I go, what could I achieve,
Trusting the hero in me?

CHORUS: *If I were brave I'd walk the razor's edge*
Where fools and dreamers dare to tread
Never lose faith, even when losing my way,
What step would I take today if I were brave?
What would I do today if I were brave?

What if we're all meant to do what we secretly dream?
What would you ask if you knew you could have anything?
Like the might oak sleeps in the heart of a seed,
Are there miracles in you and me?

CHORUS: *If I were brave I'd walk the razor's edge*
Where fools and dreamers dare to tread
Never lose faith, even when losing my way,
What step would I take today if I were brave?
What would I do today if I were brave?
What would I do today if I were brave?

If I refuse to listen to the voice of fear,
Would the voice of courage whisper in my ear?

CHORUS: *If I were brave I'd walk the razor's edge*
Where fools and dreamers dare to tread
Never lose faith, even when losing my way,
What step would I take today if I were brave?
What would I do today if I were brave?
What would I do today if I were brave?

Table of Contents

Table of Contents

$\mathscr{T}$able of $\mathscr{C}$ontents

GREETINGS!

You hold in your hands a book that we like to envision as a doorway to the philosophy and heart of the Speaking of Women's Health mission. We invite you to enter and enjoy the visit!

The mission of Speaking of Women's Health is "to educate women to make informed decisions about their health, well-being and personal safety."

From the day of its inception, Speaking of Women's Health has launched dozens of exciting programs and initiatives but never strayed from its primary goal: Give women the sound and personal health information they need to make informed choices about their lives and the lives and health of those who are close to them.

This book is chock full of information, tips, advice and thought starters to help you focus on the topics and health challenges that are most important to you. It will help you become a better-informed woman, wife, mother, daughter, sister and friend. It will enhance your level of communication and interaction with your doctor and health care professionals, so that you make the important decisions that are best for you and your loved ones. Mostly, it will lead to a healthier, more vital you.

Lots of the gadgets and devices we use in our daily lives arrive with spiffy maintenance manuals, diagrams, how-to lists and troubleshooting tips. But the human body, unfortunately, does not come with instructions. Sometimes we learn about our own health as a result of self-discovery and sheer inquisitiveness. Sometimes, a sudden emergency or unexpected health challenge sends us on a crash course to find out everything possible about a certain health problem or condition. Sometimes, we learn to help those around us, and sometimes we learn because we want to stay current and continue living full, meaningful and determined lives.

Think of this book as a doorway to Speaking of Women's Health and the powerful women and sponsors who make it possible. Please turn each page as if you're entering a new room filled with reassurance, information and guidance. Consider this book as a friend who escorts you and helps you find your way. This isn't a substitute for good health care, just a companion that will join you and your health care team on the journey.

Keeping up-to-date with the latest health trends, research studies and findings is quite a challenge. Sometimes, information and research change on a daily basis. Often, yesterday's tried-and-true recommendations become tomorrow's retractions, and as women, caregivers and patients, we're left to wonder what's right for us.

With this book, we hope to provide sound, basic information that serves as a platform for you to maintain perspective, figure out what you need for YOU and forge ahead with the knowledge you need to continue searching, asking and finding the solutions that work for you. As always, good communication between you and your health care team should always determine your plan of action, and we encourage you to use this information to help cement and deepen your relationships and ability to communicate with the people you trust for professional health advice and care.

Spend as much or as little time as you need with this book. Read it one chapter at a time. Use it for quick reference. Come back for future visits, consult it again when your life situation evolves and changes, and consider bringing your friends along, too. Use our web site as a companion to this book; giving you access to information that is constantly being updated. Visit as often as you like at **www.speakingofwomenshealth.com**. Check out our special section, called Expressly My Health. There you will find the most current information on issues important to you and your family.

Everyone can use the help of a friend to travel through life, and we want you to consider this book a companion on life's journey. Travel well!

Best,
The Staff at
Speaking of Women's Health

This book is designed to provide information about health, not medical advice. Please consult your physician if you have any questions or concerns.

CHAPTER 1

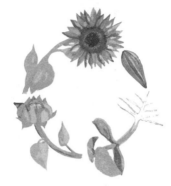

HEALTHY RELATIONSHIPS

Building a health care team is like creating a wonderful meal – you need the best ingredients possible, a plan or recipe, the proper tools to cook with, and people around you to share the feasts of your efforts. Let's look at some of the ingredients for maintaining health and well-being for you and your family: friends, doctors/health care providers, pharmacists, family and informational resources. Staying healthy is an individual endeavor that loves company!

FRIENDS

All humans have a natural need for friends, and for good reason. Friends can help increase enjoyment of life. The presence of friends can ward off feelings of loneliness, depression and low moods. People who have plenty of friends often have more outlets for talking about or reducing stress, anxiety and fears.

And increasingly, researchers are finding that the emotional support derived from friends, colleagues, spouses and others can be powerful medicine.

Women seem to know that intuitively. They routinely help each other through life's ups and downs – the birth of a child, serious illnesses, special life events such as graduations or weddings, and difficulties such as surgery, divorce or death of a loved one. Women seek out friends and spouses because they know how much better they feel when they're connected.

As we said, studies also have found that healthy relationships have a positive impact on health in general. Solid relationships, for example, can lower the risk of heart disease and depression, and having a solid partnership can make it easier for one person to stick to a healthy diet, exercise program or a commitment to quit smoking.

The question is...WHY?

Scientists have long understood that when we're under stress, our bodies produce hormones known to suppress immune response and raise blood pressure. We've seen that those with emotional and social support from friends and loved ones have more functional immune systems, lower blood pressure, and a brain that reacts less to stressors.

The study also noted that participants who had strong social ties were 80% more likely to live longer than their peers with no social ties.

Groups, such as the non-profit Wellness Community, provide support to people nationwide fighting to survive cancer. Such groups have shown that involvement in a support group – even an online support group via computer – enjoy a healthier outlook and improved mental health benefits compared to people who try to brave diseases on their own.

So...embrace life with good friends and a loving partner. Do what you can to bolster the friendships and social networks that provide the safety net in your life:

❋ Make friends a habit. Schedule regular events with friends and stick to the schedule.

- Use technology to connect with friends as well, including e-mails, chat groups, instant messaging and the like.

- Try something traditional. Send a greeting card with a hand-written message, write a letter to a friend or keep a journal for yourself. Here's a fun suggestion for journaling...share your journal with a special friend. You keep it for a week and reflect on your feelings and thoughts, then let your friend do the same for the next week. Imagine the memories you'll create.

- Consider unique ways to spend time together, such as a day trip or special outing.

- Initiate support for yourself. Make your house or apartment the gathering spot for friends, family and loved ones.

DOCTOR-PATIENT

As a Can-Do woman, it's important to know who to call and when to call them. Women tend to make most of the decisions about health care – for themselves and their families – whether it's picking the family doctor or practitioner, evaluating health insurance plans or shopping for the right cough medicine.

It's also important to line up the best health care team that you can so that you feel confident about the decisions you make and about the people whose reputation, skills, integrity and bedside manner you trust, appreciate and depend on.

As in all good relationships, communication is critical to success.

Good communication means you have the ability to screen and choose a health care team that's right for you.

Good communication means you can talk openly, honestly and without fear of embarrassment or misunderstanding from your doctor.

Good communication means you can explore all available options and, ultimately, choose the best course of action for you.

HEALTHY RELATIONSHIPS

Picking a doctor

The biggest hurdle is finding a doctor, whether it's a family physician, an internist, a surgeon, an obstetrician-gynecologist or other kind of specialist.

Dr. Gail Carlson, health education specialist for the University of Missouri-Columbia, offers these tips for choosing a doctor the first time around, or if you're unhappy with the doctor you're currently seeing, finding a new doctor.

* First, call your health insurance plan or managed care plan and get a list of doctors who are approved providers. (NOTE: If you choose a doctor who's not on your plan's list, you'll typically have to pay more).

* Ask basic questions of yourself. Do you want a family doctor or a specialist? Do you want a doctor who practices on his/her own, or would you rather be part of a larger group practice, where doctors typically share responsibilities or fill in for each other during vacations and days off?

* Does gender matter? Do you want a male or female doctor? If you're choosing a doctor for the whole family, will your spouse or children prefer a male or female doctor? If you have teenagers, what will **THEIR** preferences be?

* Ask family members, neighbors, friends, co-workers and other people you trust for recommendations. Who **DO** they recommend? Who would they **NOT** recommend?

* Check the doctor's credentials. Is she or he a specialist? Check with the American Board of Medical Specialists to see if the doctor is indeed certified in the specialty he or she claims.

* Make a call and a visit to the doctor's office. How friendly is the operator, receptionist or person who answers the phone? How attentive are they to your questions or concerns? Are they hurried or willing to listen? Is the office clean and well staffed? Are sick patients (especially children) kept separately in the waiting room?

6

⊛ Set up an interview with the doctor – a time to meet each other and assess whether you think you can work with this doctor. Ask pertinent questions about the big topics – philosophies, education, approaches to care, diligence about keeping updated with the latest medical developments, openness to alternative treatments, etc. – any topic that's important to YOU. And don't forget to ask the seemingly small questions, too. What are the doctor's office hours? Weekend policies? How are emergencies handled? Does the doctor return phone calls on a daily basis?

⊛ Ask about other key components of your health care team. At which hospital does the doctor have privileges? Who fills in when the doctor is on vacation?

Once you've done your homework, take time to think about how you FEEL about your encounters with the doctors you've met, because this is where you'll find your decision. Were you pleased with the interaction? Did you feel comfortable with the doctor's qualifications but turned off by his or her personality? Did he or she explain things in terms you could understand, or was communication difficult? Did the doctor present several approaches to treating a problem in a manner that would help you decide what to do? Was the doctor supportive of your ideas and philosophies about health, and did he or she view you as an important partner in your health care? Did the doctor make you feel comfortable about seeking a second opinion from another physician?

If you feel comfortable with the doctor's expertise AND ability to interact as a person, you'll be much closer to a decision.

After you've established a relationship with a doctor you trust and feel comfortable with, remember that maintaining your health is a two-way relationship. Partner with your doctor to find the most accurate, up-to-date information, tests, diagnoses and advice.

That means you have to be willing to talk about embarrassing or potentially troubling issues, whether it's about your sexual activities, bowel movements, drug use or something as difficult as domestic abuse or violence in the family.

Try, as much as possible, to keep lines of communication open. That doesn't mean swamping your doctor's office with phone calls once a day. It means being realistic about your needs and your doctor's needs. It means being open and honest with yourself, and being willing to listen to what the doctor recommends.

A KEY MEMBER OF THE TEAM: THE PHARMACIST

Many people spend a lot of energy choosing their doctor but don't think twice about where they fill a prescription. Having a trusted, competent pharmacist is a critical piece of the health care puzzle. In addition to choosing a pharmacy that has easy access for you, remember, when you have your prescription filled, you want to be able to ask your pharmacist questions. So establish a relationship with him or her, also.

"A lot of times, people can have more contact with a pharmacist than they can with a doctor, because a pharmacist is just generally more accessible," says Karen Froendhoff, a registered pharmacist at Wal-Mart. "We've been in the trenches where the people are. We know what it's like to stand in line and be sick, and I think we bring quite a balance to the health care team."

Likewise, choosing a pharmacist helps coordinate the information about the drugs that are prescribed for you and the treatments you choose. Most pharmacies now have databases that keep track of all of your prescriptions, including side effects, benefits, risks, possible interactions and the like. Having a central place where that information is stored – and a trusted professional who can guide you when you have questions or concerns – not only increases your overall chances of staying healthy but adds a needed level of assurance that you'll avoid potentially deadly drug reactions and side effects.

In the last several decades, Froendhoff adds, increased consumer interest in and demand for herbal products, alternative treatments, vitamin and mineral supplements and the like have forced pharmacists not only to stock whole new lines of products, but also to educate themselves on benefits, risks, side effects and options. So people who are interested in pursuing alternative or complementary health care often start by gathering information from the pharmacist and then taking it to their doctor, she says.

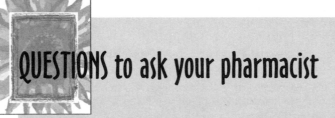

QUESTIONS to ask your pharmacist

- How often should I take this medicine? Does three times a day mean morning, noon and night, or every 8 hours around the clock?

- Should I take it on an empty stomach or not?

- What should I do if I miss a dose? Wait until the next scheduled dose or double up?

- How soon should I start to notice a difference in how I feel?

- What are possible side effects from this medicine?

- If I'm taking other medicines, vitamins or herbal supplements (tell the pharmacist exactly what they are), am I at risk for drug interactions?

- Are there certain foods or beverages that I should NOT take with this medicine or are there activities I should avoid?

HEALTHY RELATIONSHIPS

Let's talk about knowing who to call, and when. Here are 10 tips from two nurses from Bethesda North and Good Samaritan hospitals in Cincinnati, Ohio – Sharon Kowatch and Susan Wenn.

1. It is important to establish a relationship with a health care practitioner before you become ill. You need to be comfortable talking to your practitioner about all your physical and/or emotional needs.

2. It is imperative that you are well versed on your insurance coverage. Know what services/visits are covered and what are not.

3. In a true emergency situation, such as chest pain, difficulty breathing, or a severe allergic reaction, you should call 911. You need to be seen in an emergency room.

4. Ear pain and eye pain should be seen by a primary care practitioner within 24 hours of onset because serious problems can develop rapidly.

5. If you have a common flu or cold, it may not be necessary to see your practitioner, unless you have a persistent fever or the symptoms last for more than 7-10 days. Remember, antibiotics do not help because most colds and the flu are caused by a virus.

6. Many medical conditions require ongoing follow-up. Usually this is from a primary care practitioner. Some of these include diabetes, thyroid disorders, high blood pressure and cardiovascular disease. Other medical conditions that need to be evaluated include seizures, recurrent dizziness, frequent headaches, numbness of an extremity, abnormal bleeding (besides menses) and lingering pain, such as back pain, lasting more than a week.

7. It is important to be involved with the coordination and continuity of your own health care. Assist your primary care doctor or OB/GYN practitioner by bringing copies of any previous records that you may have when you see your health care provider.

8. Primary health care may be provided by physicians or by advanced practice registered nurses, such as Certified Nurse-Midwives and/or nurse practitioners. Nurse midwives and nurse practitioners diagnose and treat medical conditions and may prescribe medications in collaboration with physicians.

9. A Certified Nurse-Midwife (CNM) is a health care practitioner that has graduated from a nationally accredited program and has passed a national certification examination. CNMs provide care to women who are pregnant, seeking preventative health services or peri/postmenopausal care. Nurse-midwifery care focuses on maintaining health and encouraging women to make informed decisions about their health care.

10. A Certified Nurse Practitioner (CNP) is a health care practitioner that has advanced practice education in the field of primary care and clinical training in a health care specialty area. CNPs are also nationally certified in their specialty area and are recognized as excellent health care practitioners.

TALKING TO MEN ABOUT HEALTH

As women, we often say, "Oh, that's a guy thing, they just won't go to the doctor." We can't afford to joke about this. We need to find a way to communicate with the men in our lives about their health.

In general, as Dr. Walter Smitson, Ph.D., Professor, Department of Psychiatry, University of Cincinnati Medical Center, President & CEO, Central Clinic, Inc., says, men, unlike women, are likely to go into the "tall grasses" and wait to heal. They usually don't want to talk about their illnesses. When this happens, women may feel rejected or unvalued. We have to respect the different styles of communication between men and women. While respecting these differences, we would like to change the way men view their health. Because, according to The Men's Health Network, the ratio of male mortality over female mortality has increased in every age category for the last 30 years.

Men suffer from chronic diseases that they ignore until late in the game, when treatment is less successful and full recovery is not assured. Men who ignore routine checkups – and many do – may not know they have underlying high blood pressure, diabetes, heart disease, prostate or colon cancer, skin cancer, etc., and they pay the price with their health – and so do the women and children in their lives.

Because women tend to make most of the health care decisions, they have the opportunity to "encourage" their sons, fathers, husbands, uncles, grandfathers and friends to not only pay attention to their health, but to seek the medical care they need.

And that's not always easy.

Women need to be thoughtful about how we encourage men to take an active role in their health. These tips from the Men's Health division of ABC News provide some good guidelines for showing you care without being viewed as a nag or overbearing.

HEALTHY RELATIONSHIPS

- **Know your purpose.** If you suspect health problems, or know that a male close to you is clearly having health problems, figure out THE single most important reason to bring up the issue. Once you know the purpose, it'll be easier to approach the topic, because you'll be able to stay focused.

- **Understand his condition.** Once you've convinced the man in your life to see a doctor, learn all you can about whatever the doctor discovers. Use your own resources – the library, the Internet (www.speakingofwomenshealth.com and click on Expressly My Health), information from support groups and the like – to educate yourself so that you can appreciate what he is facing and can offer advice and information when asked.

- **Find the right time for talks.** Find calm, stress-free times to talk when you know that neither of you will be rushed or distracted.

- **Try to put yourself in his place.** Empathy is a valued trait, and trying to put yourself in his shoes will go a long way to finding common ground for answers, solutions and decisions.

- **Help him find his motivation for tackling a problem.** Try to help him identify HIS motivation for handling the problem, seeking treatment, taking medicines, agreeing to changes and making the necessary lifestyle adjustments that meet his goal. Men can be very goal-oriented, and part of your opportunity can be to help him identify and meet those goals on his terms.

- **Remind him why you feel concerned.** Let the man in your life know that you're concerned because you have feelings for him, or memories that you want to continue to build, or reasons to keep him healthy far beyond selfish ones.

- **Actively listen.** When he talks, just listen. Don't interrupt. Don't try to give advice. Don't denigrate or make him feel foolish for speaking his mind. This is one of the times to truly practice "active listening."

✧ **Remember, it's mutual.** If you're the one who's facing a health problem or challenge, be open and honest with the man or men in your life about what you need, expect and want from them. Be specific ("I need help with the laundry." or "I need help getting the kids to school.") and be general ("I need to know that you support my decision." and "I just want you to hold me.") Remember, open communication is a two-way street.

✧ **Reward success.** If it works, do it! Everyone feels good when they accomplish something they've set out to achieve. Reward success in ways that are special to you and the man in your life. Give credit when credit's due.

Speaking To Men About Their Health™
Prevention and Screening of the Most Common Cancers in Men

TYPE OF CANCER	HIGH PREVALENCE AGE	SCREENING TEST	PREVENTION
Lung Cancer	age greater than 50	none, spiral CAT scan shows promise	no smoking vitamin E
Prostate Cancer	age greater than 45	prostate-specific antigen (PSA Test) and palpation by physician	low-fat diet vitamin E or selenium
Colon Cancer	age greater than 45	stool test for blood flexible sigmoidoscopy colonoscopy	high-fiber diet vitamin E low-fat diet
Testicular Cancer	age 25-35	direct palpation by physician regular self-exam	none
Leukemia	age greater than 50	complete blood count	avoid radiation
Throat Cancer	age greater than 50	none	no smoking
Lymphoma	age 35-50	regular exam of nodes lymph and spleen	none
Skin Cancer	age greater than 30	yearly exam of moles	avoid ultraviolet light
Pancreatic Cancer	age 50-70	none	no smoking

Taken from article written by Scott Woods, MD, M.P.H., M.Ed. in *Vibrant Life*, issue May/June 2002.

TALK TO YOUR FAMILY…FOLLOW THE GENES
Sometimes, it's not till late in life that we uncover our family's "secrets." Many of the diseases that are "in the genes" can be

prevented or treated. But…you have to have the knowledge. Don't ever forget…Knowledge is Power.

Perhaps it's a history of alcoholism or mental illness that no one has ever talked about openly. Perhaps it's diseases of previous generations – conditions such as "hardening of the arteries" or "senility" – which are now recognized as underlying heart disease or Alzheimer's Disease. Our generation now has adequate information and knowledge to deal with such problems.

In minority families, genetic disorders such as sickle cell disease are important to diagnose and treat early to avoid long-term health effects. Some topics may be considered taboo. Luckily, many support groups are forming to help minority individuals and families discuss and share their successes in dealing with conditions like breast cancer in women and prostate cancer in men. The American Cancer Society, for example, sponsors the Sisters Support Network for African-American women with breast cancer and the Man-to-Man program for African-American men with prostate cancer.

Family history is important for many reasons.

"Genetic factors, along with lifestyle factors, play a part in causing many common diseases," according to the *Complete Home Medical Guide* (1999: DK Publishing) by the American College of Physicians (ACP). The organization suggests:

* Gather as much information as possible on immediate family members: brothers, sisters and parents. If possible, track down medical information on aunts, uncles and grandparents. If possible, draw a family tree that lists medical history, lifestyle factors and causes of death for individuals within your family. Don't overlook something as simple as assessing your risk factors for osteoporosis by asking if your mother or grandmother ever broke bones, particularly a hip. And certainly, heart disease can "run in the family."

* Look for patterns in families, such as chronic disorders (diabetes, allergies, learning disorders) to determine if genetic or lifestyle factors might be involved.

FAMILY TREE

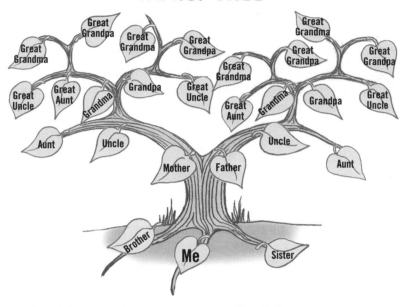

Great Grandpa · Great Grandma · Great Grandpa · Great Grandma · Great Grandpa · Great Grandpa · Great Grandma · Great Grandma · Great Uncle · Great Aunt · Grandpa · Great Uncle · Grandma · Grandpa · Great Uncle · Grandma · Great Aunt · Aunt · Uncle · Uncle · Aunt · Mother · Father · Brother · **Me** · Sister

✽ Consider genetic testing, especially if there is a strong family history of certain inherited diseases, such as heart disease, cancer, neurological disorders and the like. Sometimes, genetic testing can indicate if you're a carrier of certain genes, a finding that can help assess your own risk of developing disorders or passing them to future generations.

No matter what you find, talk openly and honestly in your family. If there's a history of alcoholism, depression, cancer, heart disease or learning disorders, for example, children need to know what they're up against. They need to know warning signs and symptoms, and they need to know what kinds of lifestyle changes they need to make to cope as well as possible or to avoid the likelihood of developing certain disorders. Why not give them the best chance possible to create healthier lives for themselves and future generations?

Staying healthy is an individual endeavor that loves company! Remember, some of the ingredients for maintaining health and well-being for you and your family: friends, doctors/health care professionals, pharmacists, family history and information resources.

CHAPTER 2

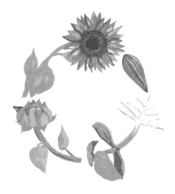

EXERCISE
There is a "Magic Medicine"

Don't you often wish there was a pill or *something* you could take that would help you feel peppier, lose weight, ward off the prospect of heart disease and osteoporosis, maintain a healthy blood pressure level, help you sleep better AND keep you younger looking?

There is.

It's called **EXERCISE!**

Before you run for the door, or begin having flashbacks to unsuccessful ventures in gym class, stop for a moment and re-think your definition of exercise.

Plainly put, exercise means activity. It means movement. It means doing something physical that gets your heart pumping and makes you break out into a sweat. If your body is doing either of those, you're exercising! (Remember, before automobiles, modern appliances, elevators and computers, human beings moved around A LOT every single day).

So let's talk first about what you can DO that counts as exercise, because you might be surprised at how little effort is involved in getting an exercise program started. You might even be surprised at how active you already are today!

"The easiest thing for women to do to get started is to do something you like," says Becky Singleton, an exercise physiologist and owner of Urban Fitness in Milton, Mass. "Think back to what you liked to do as a child. Did you like dancing? Riding your bike? Roller skating? No matter what it was, start thinking of how to incorporate that into your life today. If you like to dance, you can do that in the privacy of your own home by putting on a CD and just dancing around. Then, when you start to have fun, start looking for other activities you might like. Things like yoga, Pilates and kickboxing – none of those were part of your gym when you were growing up, so be adventurous! If you find something to do that's fun, you'll do it."

According to the *Johns Hopkins Family Health Book* (1999; HarperCollins) and the U.S. Surgeon General's office, a "moderate amount of physical activity" means burning about 150 calories a day, or about 1,000 calories a week.

A simple definition of exercise

Activity has three elements – duration (how many minutes do you exercise?), **intensity** (how hard do you work at it?) and **frequency** (how often do you do it?) By that definition, here's what "moderate" activity could involve:

- ⌇ Washing and waxing a car or washing windows/floors for 45-60 minutes
- ⌇ Playing volleyball for 45 minutes
- ⌇ Gardening for 30-45 minutes
- ⌇ Wheeling yourself in a wheelchair for 30-40 minutes
- ⌇ Walking 1.75 miles in 35 minutes
- ⌇ Bicycling 5 miles in 30 minutes
- ⌇ Dancing fast or raking leaves for 30 minutes
- ⌇ Doing water aerobics for 30 minutes
- ⌇ Pushing a stroller 1.5 miles in 30 minutes
- ⌇ Running 1.5 miles in 15 minutes
- ⌇ Stair-walking for 15 minutes

EXERCISE: There is a "Magic Medicine"

See? You already do a lot of these things. And there are many more options – rollerblading, mall walking, softball, water workouts, swimming, ballroom dancing, basketball, jumping rope, weight-lifting and yoga.

The real key is to make exercise a regular part of your life and do something that you enjoy. Ideally, you should do something physically active every day, or at least 3-4 times a week.

WHY EXERCISE?

The benefits of exercise are many, according to the American Council on Exercise. People who exercise regularly:

- Maintain a healthy body weight.
- Effectively control the pain and joint swelling of arthritis.
- Maintain lean muscle, which is often lost as one gets older.
- Have higher levels of self-esteem, self-confidence and well-being.
- Stay mentally alert and physically active longer in life.
- Reduce their risk of heart disease, high blood pressure, osteoporosis and bone loss, diabetes, high cholesterol and certain forms of cancer.
- Are mentally sharper and sleep better.

In addition, exercise has tremendous emotional benefits, including better moods, less depression or depressive thinking, more energy and less tension or anxiety. For women trying to kick a mood problem or addictive behavior like smoking or overeating, exercise is the perfect "replacement" habit. Exercise replaces the negative with a positive, and the long-term effects are far more enriching!

Three types of exercise

A complete fitness program includes three components, according to the American Council on Exercise. They are:

Aerobic exercise, or any activity that uses large muscle groups in a continuous, rhythmic fashion for sustained periods of time, enough to get the heart and lungs working and pumping. Need some examples? Running and jogging in place is considered aerobic activity. A fitness or dance class at the gym, Y or community center is aerobic. Rollerblading, dancing, playing volleyball, swimming...any activity that keeps the heart and lungs working consistently is considered aerobic, because the activity pumps oxygenated blood throughout your body.

Muscular strength and endurance conditioning, such as calisthenics, free weights or weight-lifting machines that challenge all major muscle groups – arms, chest, back, stomach, hips and legs. These types of weight-bearing exercises are especially important for maintaining the health and density of your bones, and for women, healthy bones mean you're preventing the development of osteoporosis.

A strength or conditioning program doesn't require a set of dumbbells in the basement. You can use some simple hand weights or heavy items around the house – a camera, a smooth rock, even a can of soup or fruit – and go through a simple routine of lifting them over your head, out to your side, while you do some standing squats. Take a walk and strap some ankle weights on before you head out. Sit-ups, push-ups, deep knee bends, yoga stretches and the like can all be considered strength and endurance exercises.

Flexibility means stretching that involves all major muscle groups. Before and after each workout, make sure that you stretch well and hold a mild stretch 10-30 seconds. Start simple. Bend at the waist and let your arms drop toward the floor. Hold the pose for 20-30 seconds, bending a little lower with each deep breath. Do standing stretches, making sure to reach arms and hands outward and upward for prolonged poses, and be sure to hold it more than a few seconds. As with strength conditioning, try to stretch all major muscle groups and areas of the body.

EXERCISE: There is a "Magic Medicine"

Really FEEL the muscles and underlying tissue loosen up and stretch out as you try different poses and techniques. A simple stretching book or yoga book will help you get started.

Before you start...

As always, check with your doctor before you begin an "official" exercise program, especially if you've been inactive up until now and if you have any underlying health problems or risks (if you're over 40, have risk factors for heart disease, if you smoke, are diabetic, pregnant or have suffered injuries in the past).

When choosing to exercise, do what you like. If you're going to do it, you might as well have fun, right? For the ideal workout, consider "cross training," which simply means you mix up your workouts and do several different things on different days of the week, just to keep your activities varied, challenging and non-boring. For example, you can exercise to a 40-minute videotape on Monday, take a 30-minute walk with a friend on Wednesday, attend a yoga class on Friday and maybe squeeze in a swim or a bike ride on Sunday. Exercise doesn't have to be the same thing all the time. Remember, the key is to find what you enjoy doing and do it!

WEIGHT LOSS? IT'S A BENEFIT, NOT THE GOAL

Pay attention to more than the scale or the measurement of your waistline, Singleton says. Some women begin an "exercise program" because they want to lose weight, but exercising is about far more than shedding a few pounds, she says. In fact, some people exercise regularly and still don't lose all the weight they want. But because of the exercise in their lives, they're far healthier than people who don't do anything physical.

"Exercise is what's good for you and your body," Singleton says. "Exercise is something that everybody should be doing, no matter what age. Our bodies were meant to *move*."

The whole point of exercise is to improve your health, to stave off problems that come from inactivity and to feel better.

So pay attention to how you feel after you exercise – your mood, your ability to think clearly, your level of energy, your zest for life.

Chances are, once you start, you won't be able to stop...or if you do, you'll notice that your body wants you to start again!

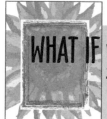

WHAT IF you're overweight and feel too embarrassed to exercise?

"People always think they have to go to a gym to exercise, and that's not always true," Singleton points out. "It all goes back to changing your mind about what you view as exercise. Beginning is always the hardest, but once you start feeling better, then it becomes the norm. The real test is consistency over time."

Start small. Buy a new pair of walking shoes and walk around the block every night. That's 10 minutes of exercise. Once that feels normal, "10 minutes turns into 20 minutes and that turns into 30 minutes, and that's exercise," she says.

Buy a CD or videotape and get moving in the privacy of your own home. If you're self-conscious about walking or pursuing some exercise outside, get up earlier than everyone else in the neighborhood and get moving when no one's watching.

"We can't let fears and self-consciousness about exercise paralyze us," Singleton says. "We need to exercise every day, the same as we brush our teeth every day. At every age, every person needs to hear that. The earlier you learn it, the better it will be for you. Your body is meant to move every day, and you can do it."

THE CORRECT GEAR

First of all, you don't need expensive clothing or perfect weather to exercise. Inclement weather shouldn't stop you. A little rain? Some snow? A hot day? So what...Be prepared for weather, and you'll be prepared for exercise.

EXERCISE: There is a "Magic Medicine"

Dress appropriately. Affordable exercise gear can be found almost anywhere. Wear lightweight clothing that breathes and allows sweat to evaporate. Some women prefer a simple cotton T-shirt and shorts, because it absorbs perspiration. Once you are really "into" exercising, you may want to consider combination fabrics made specifically for exercise. Blended fabrics that allow perspiration to "wick away" from the body are a great choice (same goes for socks).

In winter, dress in layers so that you can remove layers as your body heats up but put them back on when you cool down. Wear a supportive bra to avoid breast discomfort.

When exercising outdoors at dawn or dusk, be sure to wear reflective strips on your clothing, shoes or on your exercise equipment.

Drink plenty of water, and take it with you if you're running, biking or moving somewhere where it might not be available.

Stretch beforehand, stretch afterward. Stretching increases blood circulation to the muscles and tissues, and it flushes out the byproducts of muscular activity – substances like lactic acid – that can cause soreness and pain the next day. Stretching also strengthens muscle and tissue, making it more available to do hard work and less prone to a sprain, strain or pull.

If the shoe fits....

Wear good shoes! Good shoes, appropriate for the sport or activity, can make a world of difference in the results. Ill-fitting shoes can cause foot, leg, knee and hip pain, especially if they're worn out or don't have the kind of support that you need for your body type or the particular activity you're doing.

Today's shoe manufacturers make many different kinds of shoes, and your choice should depend on the type of sport or activity you're interested in and the unique characteristics of your feet.

Consider these tips from the American Academy of Orthopedic Surgeons:

* Try on shoes after a workout or at the end of the day, when blood has been circulating and pooling and your feet are the largest.

* Wear the same type of sock that you intend to wear for the sport or activity you have in mind. Always try on BOTH shoes; many people have different-sized or different-shaped feet.

* Forget about a "break-in" period. Shoes should be comfortable the minute you try them on. If not, keep looking!

* The heel should fit firmly with no slipping and you should be able to wiggle all your toes freely.

* Do your homework before shopping. Familiarize yourself with the different styles, makes and types of shoes. Do you need lots of arch support or very little? Lightweight shoes that accommodate the roll of the foot during walking or running, or sturdier shoes with a firm sole for a court sport such as volleyball or tennis?

KEEP YOUR EYE ON THE GOAL – MOVEMENT!

It pays to say it again: the human body was designed to MOVE every single day. Don't feel disappointed if you miss a workout every once in a while, but make a plan to include some type of physical activity on a regular basis. Pencil it into your planner. Mark it on the calendar. Discuss it at family meetings and don't let yourself make excuses for avoiding it or postponing it. This can be a wonderful way for you and your family to spend quality time together. There are lots of physical activities that the entire family can do…even if it's just a simple walk….it's also a great opportunity for communication. You'll be amazed what your kids may share with you during a walk or a bike ride.

Once it becomes part of your life, you won't want to give it up.

Now…don't you feel better already?

EXERCISE: There is a "Magic Medicine"

Homegrown exercise ideas

If you automatically associate "exercise" with a 40-minute sweaty workout in a gym or fitness center, you're missing the point. It's perfectly fine to schedule a 30-minute workout into your schedule four times a week, but you'll get similar benefits by exercising for 10 minutes three times a day. And you're probably already exercising, or could very easily incorporate it into your life, with a few simple lifestyle changes.

If you take the elevator at work, start taking the stairs. Walk the stairs for 10 minutes on a lunch break or at the end of the day.

When was the last time you walked to your neighborhood market? The library? Around the block with your children? A simple walk is one of the best forms of exercise, and one of the easiest to begin.

Does your home have hardwood floors? Next time you treat or wax them, use a terrycloth towel and your feet to do the buffing. Turn up the stereo full blast to get the full effect. Do the twist, boogie-woogie or any movement that feels good and gets the job done!

Get a dog! You might be able to talk yourself out of a walk every day, but a dog .... allows you no excuses! Many people find that the routine of walking a pet is a great motivation to start a walking or exercise program.

Don't just stand on the sidelines at your child's next sporting event. Find another "soccer" mom (pick your sport) and walk around the field, the school hallways, or the neighborhood during lulls in the activity.

Next time you drive to the mall or cinema, park farther away from the entrance, but in a well-lit and well-traveled area. Or, get off the train or bus a few stops early and walk the rest of the way to your destination.

24

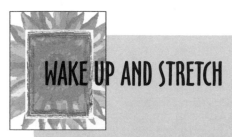

WAKE UP AND STRETCH

Here are some tips from Speaking of Women's Health experts Pam Butler, Jeanine Roth and Dorothy Mann.

Warm up first

Make sure you are working warm muscles. Do a brief 10 to 15 minute warm up, then begin your flexibility training.

Functional flexibility

Based on your daily activities, develop a flexibility program to help increase your mobility and stability as well as help you maintain proper body alignment during daily activities. For example, if you regularly sit or stand for long periods of time, or are required to bend and lift, flexibility training will help you with these activities.

Listen to your body

Pay special attention to tight areas. Shoulders, hamstrings and the lower back tend to be over-tight and may hold tension.

Do's & don'ts

Pay attention to your body's signals and don't push too far. Never use bouncing or jerking movements. Hold each stretch for 10 to 30 seconds.

Be creative and consistent

Vary your flexibility training routine. To fully benefit, integrate regular stretching into your permanent fitness routine.

CHAPTER 3

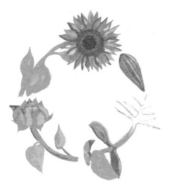

NUTRITION

As one of our experts jokes, "If I truly am what I eat, I am fast, cheap and easy!" We all laugh. But, what are we laughing about?

For many women, the daily reality of their lives is a food puzzle. Perhaps no other topic relating to health is more confusing than food and nutrition.

Women are bombarded by "miracle" diet claims and advertisements, treatments, surgical procedures and pills promising immediate weight loss and thinner bodies. They're surrounded by conflicting medical studies on food and nutrition, such that one week's hugely popular "must-have" food is tops on next week's "don't eat" list because of the ever-changing or constantly conflicting studies.

As a result, many women swing from one food fad to another, high-carbohydrate diets to high-protein diets, from fruit-heavy diets to purely pasta diets, from food supplements to macrobiotic diets – not because they can't make up their minds, but because the information they receive is conflicting, and even medical experts sometimes can't agree what's what.

And the results?

Making the Nutrition Pieces Fit

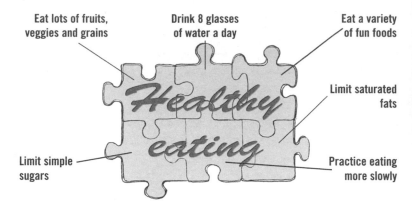

Eat lots of fruits, veggies and grains

Drink 8 glasses of water a day

Eat a variety of fun foods

Limit saturated fats

Limit simple sugars

Practice eating more slowly

As a nation, we're fatter than ever. More than one-third of all Americans are considered obese – carrying far more weight on their frames than their body type and height call for. And it's not just a problem among adults. According to the U.S. Department of Health and Human Services, 15% of children, including 10% of pre-schoolers, were considered overweight or obese in 2002.

And nutritionally, our bodies may not be getting the necessary vitamins, minerals, amino acids, proteins and nutrients they need to maintain good health and ward off the health problems that are linked to poor nutrition.

Poor health, obesity and inadequate nutrition are directly tied to choices about eating. So let's look at what's happening.

As a nation, we eat too much and exercise too little, and when we DO eat, we're eating the wrong things, in serving sizes that are far too large for the average human body, or in forms (fried vs. baked) that simply do not deliver enough nourishment to maintain health or a normal weight.

"Here's the catch," says Susan Finn, R.D., L.D. "Even though we know a lot about food and nutrition, we don't always eat the way we know we should."

Perhaps what we've forgotten is that food is a nutrient-rich

NUTRITION

fuel source for the body. Good nutrition means providing the body with all of the elements it needs – vitamins, minerals, protein, fiber, amino acids, etc. – to pump blood into and out of the heart, inflate and deflate the lungs, nourish cells, feed the brain, power the body's muscles, maintain nerve impulses and fight off disease.

What goes into each body has a dramatic effect on the health of that body. Poorly nourished bodies are at greater risk for a variety of health problems, from simple vitamin deficiencies to serious cancers, from a high risk of a heart attack to brittle fingernails, from poor pregnancy outcomes to weakened bones. Indeed, some of today's leading causes of death – cancer, heart disease, diabetes and stroke – are heavily influenced by poor nutrition and/or excessive food intake.

Women in particular need special minerals and nutrients at various times in their lives – more iron during their menstrual years, more calcium throughout life to build and maintain healthy bones, and folic acid before and during pregnancy to prevent neural tube defects in their babies, as well as for their own healthy hearts throughout life.

And the body's nutritional needs change over time. Adolescent girls need plenty of calcium to build strong bones, and many don't realize that most of the bone growth takes place by age 20. As women mature, the goal is to keep the bones as calcium-dense as possible and to stave off the inevitable leaching of calcium and minerals out of the bones that occurs in middle age and older years, putting women at risk of osteoporosis and bone fractures. (See Chapter 11)

As the body ages, metabolism slows. Older women who don't change the amount of food that they eat will nonetheless see the pounds add up, because the body is not as capable of breaking food down and using it as energy.

So, where to start with the huge topic of nutrition?

Let's start with some simple guidelines from the U.S. Department of Agriculture, and then go from there.

Simple eating guidelines

- Eat a variety of foods.
- Balance the food you eat with physical activity. Do something active 3-4 times a week for 30 minutes.
- Choose a diet with moderate amounts of salt and sodium.
- Choose a diet moderate in sugars.
- Eat plenty of vegetables, fruits and grains. Federal experts recommend at least five servings a day of fresh fruits and vegetables – raw, cooked, juices – however you can get them into your body.
- While you're working on improving your diet, if you know your eating style isn't ideal, consider a multivitamin once a day to make up for the vitamins and minerals you aren't getting from food.

With those guidelines to work from, then what?

Finn's first suggestion is simple to offer, harder to actually accomplish: SLOW DOWN!

"I think we are in a time of what we call the **hurried woman syndrome**," she says. "People are just grabbing at anything to eat. Why else would 15% of breakfasts be eaten in the car, and why are we adding so many cup holders to mini-vans? People are gulping and eating things and don't even know what they are…it's more like frantic, nervous eating. Nine times out of ten, nervous eating equals unhealthy choices. And my advice is to slow down."

How? Finn offers these tips:

- Next time you sense a feeling of stress, stop and take a deep breath. Physically and mentally slow yourself down so that you can make wise choices.

NUTRITION

* Ask yourself what's really important – the health of you and your family, or adding another chore to your to-do list? Chances are, you'll vote for your health and that of your family, and make conscious choices about what you put in your mouth and theirs.

MAKE SMALL CHANGES

"In the long run," Finn says, "small changes are really what's going to make the best improvements in the diets of women. If you set goals so big that nobody can achieve them – and that applies to eating as well as to running a business – your chances of success are less." So make the small changes, she suggests, by asking simple questions, such as: "What am I really eating?"

Keep a food diary, or consciously pay attention to what you put into your mouth over the course of a day, to get a true grip of what you're eating and in what amount. Then ask yourself: "Is that really what I want to eat? Are there better options?"

Yes, small changes can have profound effects on health, she says. If needed, losing just 5 pounds, for example, can lower blood sugar and reduce the risk of diabetes or pre-diabetic conditions. A loss of 10 pounds can lower blood pressure and cholesterol levels. As weight loss increases, so do the health benefits, such as a lower risk of certain cancers, heart disease, arthritis, high blood pressure, sleep problems and more.

Dieting, as study after study proves, simply doesn't work. People lose weight by dieting, but more than 90% of the time, people who diet gain the weight back – and then some. So if there's a new "fad diet" out there, avoid it. Like other fads, it'll go away soon when people realize it doesn't work.

The trick is to develop a lifelong eating plan that works for you. It always helps to check with your family doctor first, because you may have special nutritional needs that will rule out some kinds of diets or eating plans. If you like the philosophies of the protein-heavy and carbohydrate-restricting diets, for example, follow them if they work for you – and make sure that whatever foods you eat within its parameters are balanced and nutrient-rich. If you decide to become a vegetarian, make sure you get enough protein and vitamins typically lacking in a vegetarian diet. Whatever you decide, research your approach before you start so that you're eating smartly.

And don't punish yourself if you "slip up" or fall off your eating plan for a while. Just resolve to pick it up again and eat well – for your own good health.

FOCUS ON "GOOD-FOR-YOU" FOODS

As the rate of obesity has increased among Americans, restaurants and food manufacturers have come under fire from critics who blame the high-fat, low-nutrient value of today's fast and ready-to-eat foods for the nation's weight problem. But Finn doesn't buy that line of thinking.

"Weight gain and bad eating are not based on fast foods or what food companies offer," she says. "I believe it's what you choose, and you have to consciously make sure you put some

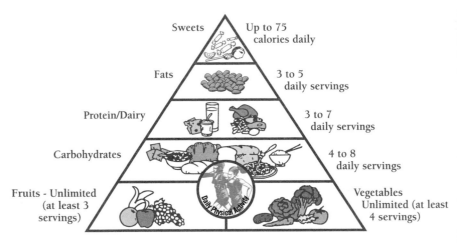

This guide aids in helping you create a balanced diet by showing you the recommended daily servings from all of the food groups.

Source: The Mayo Clinic Healthy Weight Pyramid

good-for-you foods into your diet. It can be something as simple as a wrap or some well-chosen fast foods, an energy bar or some sort of a fully balanced beverage drink."

Busy women with busy lives have plenty of options when they're hungry, she says, and it's far better nutritionally to tuck a protein shake drink or protein bar into your backpack or briefcase than it is to make a quick run through the fast-food drive-thru. Energy bars and drinks are balanced nutritionally, packed with plenty of vitamins, minerals and nutrients that quickie restaurant meals just can't provide. And they're already in the right portions, so you won't overeat or overindulge.

Take along a small bag of fresh, cut-up carrots, green peppers or broccoli florets. These, "good-for-you-foods while you're on the go, equal portion control," Finn says. "**AND PORTION CONTROL IS WEIGHT CONTROL.**"

Speaking of portion control, just say "no" to super-sizing as well.

As the nation's waistline has expanded, so has the size of the portions of food that are served in restaurants, pre-packaged goods and at home. Think back to the first cute little glass bottles of soda, introduced in the 1940s. For several decades, a 6-ounce bottle of soda was the standard size of a single soft-drink serving. Over the years, single servings have gotten larger and larger. A 54-ounce cup – a whopping nine times larger than when the first bottles were introduced – is now available at quick-stop markets. Likewise, Finn points out, a 1950s muffin weighed about 1.5 ounces, compared with a full 8 ounces for some of today's super muffins. And French fries? The first orders were about 2 ounces and had about 200 calories – compared to a 7-ounce serving today that packs a whopping 610 calories. Do we really need ALL that food and drink? Obviously not!

Finn urges women to exert portion control on their own.

Muffin 1.5 oz.

Muffin 8 oz.

- When asked to "super-size" at restaurants, politely decline.
- When served large portions, divide it into smaller portions and take home the extra in a "doggie bag."
- When ordering an entrée at a restaurant, share it with a friend.

Emotional eating...or true hunger?

It's no secret that many people turn to food when they're stressed, worried, sad, lonely or trying to cope with a range of emotional feelings. It's called "emotional hunger," meaning people use food to feel full and satisfied, even though the underlying emotional need still goes unfilled.

Consciously pay attention to when you snack. Is it at night when you watch television? At work when you're stressed? At social events where alcohol is served? When a relationship problem is weighing heavily on your mind? Pay attention to when and why you snack, and be prepared to choose healthy snacks when you feel the urge – a protein drink, for example, or a piece of fruit instead of something salty or fatty.

Limit fat and calories

Because it's the leading cause of death in women, heart disease ought to be a primary focus of women as they look at sound nutrition. 37% of the women in America will die of heart disease! You can change that statistic.

- Eat plenty of fresh fruits and vegetables, whole grains, legumes (beans, peas). Two 4-ounce servings of fish that are high in Omega-3 fatty acids (such as salmon), consumed each week can reduce your risk of heart disease.
- Avoid foods high in saturated fat, such as fatty meats. Most experts recommend a diet with no more than 20%-30% fat.
- Use olive oil, other vegetable oils or vegetable sprays for cooking.
- Choose low-fat dairy products.
- Eat foods high in fiber.

NUTRITION

Calcium

To keep bones healthy and strong – and less likely to fracture with age – get plenty of calcium. Good sources include:

- Fortified milk, yogurt and cheese
- Calcium-fortified drinks and breakfast foods
- Salmon and sardines with bones
- Canned shrimp
- Dried figs
- Cooked rhubarb
- Broccoli, collard greens, kale, turnip greens
- Soybeans, tofu
- Blackstrap molasses

Consider a calcium supplement, but talk to a dietitian or pharmacist about the best kind. Some forms of calcium are absorbed better than others, and some forms may have higher than recommended traces of heavy metals, such as lead. And remember, you also need Vitamin D (fortified cereals, egg yolks, fish oil) to absorb the calcium, Vitamin C (oranges, potatoes, cantaloupe, citrus fruits) to form the collagen that creates a matrix in your bone for calcium to build, and other trace elements and vitamins to get a complete nutrient profile. Remember, calcium is vital for strong bones, but it may not be enough to prevent osteoporosis. After menopause or at age 55, ask your doctor about having a Dexa Scan to determine your bone density. If you have osteopenia or osteoporosis, he or she may prescribe a medication to help reduce your risk for bone fractures.

Iron

Because they lose iron each month due to menstruation, women need to replenish the body's stores of iron.

Most multi-vitamin supplements with added iron are perfectly fine.

Iron is also found in red meats, chicken, fish, liver, spinach and leafy green vegetables, enriched whole grain breads and cereals, pinto beans and prunes.

Folic Acid

This mineral is important for preventing common birth defects, including spina bifida. If considering pregnancy, begin taking folic acid immediately. Prenatal vitamins contain folic acid, and so do some vitamins found at your pharmacy. The earlier you begin, the greater the chances of preventing birth defects or neural-tube defects in infants. Remember, folic acid is also essential for maintaining heart health throughout life.

Diabetes control

Diabetes occurs when your body cannot make enough insulin to control sugar levels in your blood or cannot use it properly. Insulin is a hormone that converts sugar into instant energy or body fat.

People with diabetes have the same nutritional needs as everyone else, but they can keep the disease under control. Suggestions include:

- **Maintain a healthy weight.** Obesity is a leading (and growing) cause of diabetes today.

- **Eat balanced meals** to keep blood sugar levels as close to normal as possible. Many pre-packed food bars, meals and drinks are now made specifically for people with diabetes, both to provide balanced nutrition and to limit sugar. Check with a dietitian or your doctor about the growing number of choices available to you.

- **Limit fat in the diet.** According to the Physicians Committee for Responsible Medicine, more fat in the diet makes it hard for sugars to be used by cells. Some diabetics, in fact, turn to vegetarian diets to control their disease.

- **Talk with a dietitian** to learn more about eating well to control insulin and blood sugars.

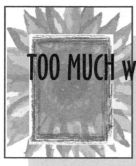

TOO MUCH weight = ill health

Health consequences linked to obesity, according to the U.S. Centers for Disease Control, include:

- High blood pressure

- High blood cholesterol

- Diabetes

- Heart disease, stroke and chest pain

- Congestive heart failure

- Gallbladder disease and gallstones

- Gout

- Osteoarthritis

- Obstructive sleep apnea (snoring/stopped breathing during sleep) and breathing problems

- Pregnancy complications

- Menstrual irregularities, infertility, irregular ovulation

- Bladder control problems (stress incontinence)

- Kidney disease

- Psychological problems, including depression, eating disorders, distorted body image and low self-esteem

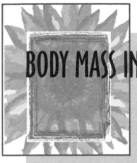

BODY MASS INDEX: Figure it Out!

The latest scale for determining a person's overall health is a measurement called the Body Mass Index. Basically, it calculates the relationship of your height to your weight, and it's more highly correlated with body fat than other body-mass measurements, according to the U.S. Centers for Disease Control.

To calculate your Body Mass Index: use this equation.

⊛ Find your weight in pounds and multiply it by 705.

⊛ Now find your height in inches, and multiply that number by itself (height squared).

⊛ Now divide the height number by your weight. That number is your Body Mass Index.

Need an example? Say you're a 130-pound woman who stands 5 feet 7 inches tall (or 67 inches total).

⊛ 130 pounds times 705 equals 91,650
⊛ 67 times 67 equals 4489
⊛ Now divide 91,650 by 4489 to get 20.4

- Individuals with a BMI under 20 are considered underweight.

- Those with a BMI of 20-25 are considered normal.

- Those with a BMI of 25-29.9 are considered overweight.

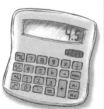

- Those with BMI of 30 or higher are considered obese.

CHAPTER 4

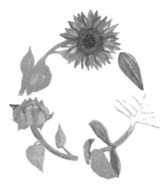

THE BEAUTIFUL YOU, INSIDE OUT

Our mothers and our grandmothers were right! Remember all the advice and one-liners they used to offer on days when we didn't feel or look so great? Or felt as if we didn't fit in? Or just needed someone to cheer us up?

"Beauty is only skin deep....It's what's on the inside that counts."

"People don't love you for your body...they love you for your mind."

"Whatever makes you special is what makes you beautiful."

Perhaps they knew what many women learn as they grow older and more mature: beauty is a combination of body and mind, appearance and soul, personality and mindset.

Some women do have a glow about them, and it may not be from sheer, knockout beauty. You may feel drawn to such women because of their self-confidence or the enthusiasm and the glow that they exude. They embrace life to the fullest.

Just as traditional medicine is paying more and more attention to the tremendous connection between physical health and mental attitude and outlook, so too is the beauty-care and self-care industry making the connection between good health and self-esteem.

And most women need a little help to look their best. Women who look good, feel better. Women who feel better take better care of themselves and pass their spirit and energy to those around them. And when you feel good about your life – what you're doing, what you're achieving, and the legacy you're passing to others – you gain the confidence and courage to face whatever life throws your way.

And who can argue with a cycle like that?

Let's take a look at some ways you can shape and create the beautiful you….from the inside out!

SKIN CARE

As the comedian George Carlin used to joke, "Skin is what keeps your insides in." But it's so much more than that! It's the largest organ in the body, a protective covering that lives and breathes, and a busy, busy place.

Just one square inch of your skin contains 1,300 nerve endings, 65 hairs, up to 100 oil glands, 650 sweat glands and 9.5 million cells. That's a lot of activity going on!

But the skin is also an indicator of the state of your health – and the first thing that other people see when they meet and look at you for the first time.

No matter what your skin tone or skin texture, no matter what your ethnic background or skin color, proper skin care is important to maintaining overall health and putting your best "you" forward.

The skin has two layers

The top layer, or **epidermis**, is what's visible to you and everyone else. In this layer, new skin cells are generated and melanin, the substance that adds color and pigment to the skin, is produced.

Underneath the epidermis is the other 90% of your skin, the **dermis**. It contains

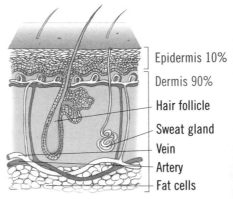

Epidermis 10%

Dermis 90%

Hair follicle

Sweat gland

Vein

Artery

Fat cells

collagen and elastin fibers that keep the skin supple, stretchy and strong. The layer is also laced with other components, including blood vessels, nerve fibers and nerve endings, oil glands, muscle cells and hair follicles.

A fat layer underneath the dermis protects, cushions and insulates the skin, and its thickness depends on your age, health, diet and amount of physical activity.

THE SKIN HAS LOTS OF JOBS TO DO:

* **It protects the body,** serving as a barrier that keeps out bacteria, infectious germs, pollution and injury.
* **It retains water,** serving as a barrier that locks in moisture throughout the body.
* **It regulates body temperature,** relying on its insulating layers to keep in heat and to cool off the body with perspiration.
* **It cleanses the body,** allowing small amounts of waste to pass out of the body in sweat.
* **It's a nerve center,** and the millions of nerve endings and fibers in the skin control our sense of touch, weight, pressure, heat, cold, pleasure, pain and movement.
* **It produces Vitamin D when exposed to sunlight,** creating a necessary vitamin that helps the body absorb calcium and phosphates from food.

Left to its own devices, skin has a lot of work to do. But like all organs, it begins to age and wear out over time, although some women live far into their 80s and 90s with healthy, vibrant skin.

That's because many habits, behaviors and lifestyle choices can affect the health and appearance of skin. Some of the lifestyle factors that can influence how your skin looks and performs include:

Alcohol: Drinking significant quantities of alcohol interferes with circulation and dries out the skin.

Cigarettes: Heat, tobacco and nicotine damage the elastic part of the skin and cause blood vessels under the skin to shrink, preventing necessary oxygen and blood flow from getting to the skin.

Crash and yo-yo diets: Rapid weight loss and the regaining of weight can stretch and shrink, stretch and shrink skin, causing it to sag over time.

Diet: Skin requires plenty of nutrients, vitamins and minerals to remain healthy. Diets high in fat and sugar do little to support what the skin needs.

Emotional health: Have you ever noticed that your face breaks out when you're upset or stressed? Or that worry can make your eyes look saggy and tired? The mind-body connection is important for skin health, too.

Exercise: Being physically active improves circulation, delivers nutrients and oxygen to the skin cells and creates new blood vessels. Sweating also flushes toxins out of the body through the skin, keeping it energized.

Skin-care products: Some skin products are harsh because they contain substances that burn, irritate, dry out or damage skin permanently. Be careful about what you put on your skin (and scalp). Read ingredients, and choose items from companies that have invested in research and development to create safe, effective products.

Sleep: They call it "beauty sleep" for a reason! When you sleep, your body is busy rejuvenating itself, building new cells and regenerating.

Sunshine and ultra-violet exposure: Perhaps no other factor can more negatively affect the long-term health and appearance of your skin. Suntans and exposure to the ultra-violet rays of sunlight are the leading causes of skin cancer, wrinkles, blotches, age spots and premature aging.

Water: Your skin needs plenty of water to stay supple and moist, and drinking water is one of the best things you can do for overall health.

THE BEAUTIFUL YOU, INSIDE OUT

Know your skin type

If everyone had the same kind of skin, the variety of skin-care products at the local cosmetics counter or pharmacy store would be far less robust than it is. It's important to know your skin type and to choose appropriate cleansers, moisturizers and cosmetics.

Basically, skin is grouped into four different types.

Normal skin is exactly what it says: normal, vibrant, well hydrated throughout and smooth. Even normal skin can react negatively to sunlight, hormones and other factors, but its overall health and appearance are good. How to care for it: Use a mild soap or facial cleansing cloth for normal skin and be sure to avoid harsh scrubs or toners that contain alcohol or other drying ingredients.

Dry skin lacks moisture and has a dry look. Dry skin can flake, look dull or appear cracked and wrinkled. Usually dry skin doesn't produce enough oil, or it's exposed to certain things – harsh products, cigarette smoke, too much sunlight, wind, even emotional stress – that make it look dried out. How to care for it: Avoid soaps or cleansers that can dry it out even further. Wash with warm water (not hot!) and a "no-detergent" facial soap. Use a good moisturizer during the day (as many times as needed) and consider a night cream that will keep it hydrated while you sleep.

Oily skin tends to appear oily or greasy, especially across the forehead and down the nose. Sometimes, the oil glands do produce too much oil. Harsh products or too much sun can make skin appear oily on the surface but the skin actually may be lacking true moisture in the deeper layers. Oily skin might have large pores, breakouts or blemishes. How to care for it: Don't overdo it! Washing or cleansing too frequently can actually spur the skin to create even more oils, compounding the problem. Cleanse it regularly, especially after exercise or vigorous activity, but don't scrub it harshly. Keep hands away from the face, remove makeup before going to bed. Oily skin is usually shiny in its appearance, especially in the T-Zone. The T-Zone is the area across the forehead and down the nose.

Combination skin means you have a little bit of both – some parts of your skin are normal, some are oily, some might even be dry. How to care for it: Cleanse your skin as you would normal skin, and pay particular attention to oily or dry areas and moisturize and cleanse them appropriately.

Daily skin care

Regardless of your skin type, daily skin care should involve four steps:

* **Cleanse the skin**, preferably at least twice a day. Use gentle, mild cleansers that do not irritate the skin. Washing the skin removes dirt, grit and grime, and cleans out the pores so that the skin can function normally.

* **Exfoliate the skin**, which means using products that rid the skin of the top layer of cells. Too much exfoliation can irritate the skin and cause redness, rashes or soreness, so do so only when necessary and test certain methods or products to find one that works for you. A rough sponge or cloth might do just fine, or you may prefer a daily disposable cleansing cloth with a built-in exfoliant product.

* **Don't forget the moisturizer!** Cleansing the skin is one thing, adding moisturizer is another critically important step. Moisturizing means applying a cream that will add a layer to the outer skin and create a barrier that keeps the skin's own moisture from evaporating. Again, learn your skin type and try several products before you find one that works for you. Drinking plenty of water – at least 8 glasses a day – also moisturizes the skin from the inside.

⊛ **Screen out the sun.** The sun's harmful ultra-violet rays affect the skin in several ways. They can damage the collagen and elastin that keep the skin supple, causing it to sag and wrinkle. Moreover, ultra-violet rays dry out the skin, cause tiny blood vessels to break (resulting in age spots) and damage the skin's immune function, making it less able to recover from burns or damage. Always apply a sunscreen or moisturizer with a Sun Protection Factor of at least 15. (SPF 15 means that if you normally burn in the sun after 10 minutes, an SPF 15 lotion will allow you to stay out 15 times longer before burning. But remember that sweating, swimming, exercise and physical activity can wash it off, so reapply frequently when outdoors). Some cosmetics now have sunscreens added, saving you the two-step process of applying sunscreen and then makeup.

Women of color

Women of color have special skin care problems and needs, and luckily the personal care industry has responded with new products in recent decades. Manufacturers now create entire lines of cosmetics – foundations, powders, blushes, eye shadows, etc. – for women of color whose skin tones are dark, olive or blended.

Each skin type, in fact, has its own characteristics:

Afro-Caribbean Skin tends to be thicker, has good elasticity and healthy levels of oil, and tends to age slowly.

Asian Skin is slightly thicker than **Caucasian Skin** and because it has lots of melanin, ages slowly.

Latin Skin texture and color vary considerably and tends to be oily.

And regardless of the coloring or amount of pigment in the skin, women of color are reminded to add sunscreen to their daily routines, because skin cancer affects all shades of skin. White skin is more prone to skin cancer, but dark skin is also at risk for developing cancers.

Makeup Tips

There's plenty of variety in how women use makeup. Some don't wear it at all, or only on special occasions, while some women won't venture out without it.

Whatever your preference or lifestyle, keep in mind these simple tips about makeup:

- Know what is good for you and good for your skin. Determine what type of skin you have – normal, oily, combination or sensitive – before choosing products.
- Always remove makeup before going to bed!
- Never apply fresh makeup over old makeup. Always start with clean skin, not only for better results, but also for cleaner, healthier skin!
- Before applying makeup, make sure it has a Sun Protection Factor of 15 or higher and if not, add some sunscreen under your eyes and on your cheeks, neck and throat.
- Replenish your makeup regularly. In fact, start to think about your makeup – foundation, powders, blushes, and mascaras – as you do those old containers of food in the back of the fridge. If you don't remember what they are, or when you bought them – throw them out! If it smells, clumps, or is older than six months, pitch it! If you wouldn't consider putting old, outdated food in your mouth, why would you consider putting old, outdated makeup on your face, your window to the world?

HAIR CARE

Many women feel that their hair is one of the most important identifiers, the one thing that makes them unique or stylish. In fact, when surveyed, women in America named six signs that they identified as "healthy hair". These signs include hair that is strong, shiny, soft, silky, less frizzy and full of body.

Maybe that's why they spend so much time preparing it, fussing over it, shampooing it, conditioning it and shaping it in ever-changing and stylish ways.

Washing hair regularly to keep it clean, conditioning it to keep it lush and moisturized, and not exposing it to harsh chemicals or harsh environments can go a long way to keeping a healthy head of hair. Ingredients like panthenol, have been used to add health and shine to hair for years. In fact, panthenol is now being used in some skin care products.

Like the Judy Collins song "Paradise," hair is one of those things in life that you don't know what you've got till it's gone. And while women would love to keep their hair for a lifetime, hair does eventually thin out as women age, in some more than others, and hair loss from any cause can be traumatic for women. In fact, 25% of all women experience hereditary hair thinning, even though most of us think that hair loss only affects men. There is something that can be done, but as with most things, early treatment is most effective.

First, it's important to know that hair is always growing, always falling out, and always replenishing itself. According to the Women's Institute for Fine and Thinning Hair, the scalp loses up to 150 hairs a day, every day – a sign that the hair follicles from which individual hairs grow are resting.

For women, the hair is at its thickest at age 20, and begins to thin gradually throughout the rest of life. Women who start with a full head of thick hair may never notice the thinning process, while those whose hair is naturally thin and fine may notice it more than ever. In fact, women with thin hair tend to experience far more hair loss as they move through life than women who have full or thick hair.

What causes hair loss?

Very common conditions – pregnancy, certain medications, diets, and stress – can cause hair to thin and fall out. Some of it is natural, and hair growth will return to normal after a time.

But a condition called "alopecia" is a common hair loss disorder, and it means that the hair falls out, leaving bald patches or spots where hair refuses to grow. Sometimes it develops because of an illness or stress, or as a reaction to a medicine you're taking. If your hair growth does not return to normal, talk to your doctor about possible causes and treatments.

Hair loss can happen in women of all ethnic backgrounds. In fact, African-American women who use hair reshaping products – relaxers, straighteners, hot combs and the like – can experience what the Women's Institute for Fine and Thinning Hair calls "Traumatic Alopecia." Alopecia means loss of hair, and traumatic alopecia occurs suddenly.

African-American women who experience hair problems should consult with a stylist or dermatologist to determine the cause of hair loss and follow these recommendations to keep it from worsening or to prevent it from recurring:

- Apply chemicals to the hair, not the scalp. Try using "mild" versions of relaxers and get touch-ups less frequently.
- Use loose wrappings to minimize tension and not pull on the hair roots.
- Try braids that are larger and loose, and unbraid hair every two weeks.
- Use hair products that contain glycerin, instead of mineral oil or petroleum.
- Try hair extensions that don't require the daily stress of braiding, but avoid using glue to attach hair extensions.

Managing and treating hair loss

Hair loss can be treated, either with medicines that spur hair to grow again or by cosmetic and styling approaches that lessen its evidence.

- Talk to your stylist about a wig or hairpiece to cover the bald spot or scalp.
- Ask your stylist about a different cut or hairstyle that can cover or hide areas where hair refuses to grow. Sometimes a simple change in how your hair is cut can make all the difference in the world.
- If you wear your hair pulled back, or in a ponytail or braid, avoid tension on the roots.
- Shampoo hair gently and massage the scalp lightly to stimulate blood circulation to the hair follicles.
- Add a little conditioner to the ends of your hair after showering, but avoid all-over conditioning because it can make the hair heavier and make it look greasy.

❋ When blow drying hair, avoid high heat settings and consider drying it with a towel first to remove excessive moisture.

❋ Try products made specifically for fine or thin hair (read labels).

❋ Hair transplant surgery is an option, but as with all surgical procedures, ask plenty of questions, consider risks and benefits, compare the different types of transplant surgery and always get a second opinion.

❋ Ask your doctor about prescription drugs and over-the-counter preparations including minoxidil, that may reverse the thinning process and help stimulate hair growth.

HEALTHY SMILES

When you smile at the world, does it smile back at you?

Let's hope so, because a healthy smile can make all the difference in how women look and in how they feel – about themselves, their worth and their value to the world.

There's a direct correlation between healthy teeth and self-esteem, not to mention growing evidence that healthy teeth and gums can mean overall physical health. In fact, a growing body of evidence suggests that the bacteria that hide in the mouth in people with gum disease might actually contribute to a variety of health problems throughout the body – heart disease, diabetes, respiratory problems, premature births and more. The thinking is that the bacteria that cause gum disease enter the bloodstream directly in the gums, setting up inflammation, infections or disease elsewhere in the body.

That's why regular dental care is still recommended for children and adults. Cavities may not be the problem they once were, but overall dental health has far-reaching effects on self-esteem, overall health and a positive outlook on life.

Some dental care tips:
❋ Brush and floss daily.

❋ Get a regular dental checkup at least twice a year.

❋ Have teeth cleaned professionally at least once a year.

Be on the lookout for signs of gum disease, and see your dentist or a gum specialist if they occur. Symptoms include red, swollen or tender gums that may bleed during brushing; gums that have pulled away from the teeth; persistent bad breath; gaps between the teeth and gums; loose and separating teeth; and a difference in the way your teeth fit together when you bite, or a change in how your dentures fit.

Cosmetic dentistry: a lifesaver for dull, broken teeth

Don't be embarrassed by broken, discolored or uneven teeth. According to the American Academy of Cosmetic Dentistry, a variety of products and procedures can improve the look, function and brightness of teeth.

Discolored, stained or dull teeth: Tooth whitening, once available only in a dentist's office or under a dentist's care, can now be done with over-the-counter products that may include clear strips containing a whitening gel, which are worn on the teeth several times a day for several weeks. Professional tooth bleaching by a dentist is always an option, and although it's more expensive, it's also quicker (2-3 weeks instead of up to 6 weeks with over-the-counter products). Whatever you choose, read and follow directions carefully, because the chemicals in bleaches and whiteners can irritate the gums and cause sensitive teeth.

Chipped, cracked or worn teeth: Cosmetic dentists can restore broken teeth with thin veneers made of porcelain or composites, or through bonding, a process in which an enamel-like material is applied to the surface, sculpted, hardened and then polished.

Missing teeth or bite problems: Fixed bridges, crowns or dental implants can replace missing teeth or fill in noticeable gaps. Likewise, porcelain and ceramics can be shaped and colored to fill in missing teeth. Many adults are increasingly turning to orthodontics (braces) to take care of crooked teeth, bite problems and jaw problems. Today's newer braces are far less noticeable, and some can be worn on the backs instead of the fronts of teeth.

THE BEAUTIFUL YOU, INSIDE OUT

*It's never too late to brush up on the proper technique!
Use an electric toothbrush the same way you would
use a regular toothbrush.*

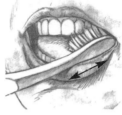

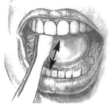

A.) Aim brush at 45 degree angle to the gum line. Use a back and forth motion, brushing in short strokes.

B.) Brush the chewing surfaces of your teeth.

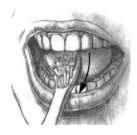

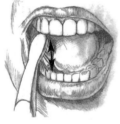

C.) Clean the inside surfaces of your teeth by brushing from the gum to the biting edge of both upper and lower teeth.

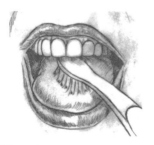

D.) To avoid bacteria and bad breath, brush the tongue.

Remember - when you smile at the world,
the world will smile back at you!

CHAPTER 5

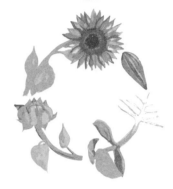

MENOPAUSE
Bring on the Change

Maybe menopause is sometimes referred to as "The Change" because that's really all it is...a change in life that, like the other cyclical ebbs and flows of a woman's life, brings a new set of challenges and issues to think about, consider and manage.

For some women, menopause is a big deal. For others, it's a barely noticeable shift from the child-bearing years into years of "post-menopausal zest" and discovery.

Since the beginning of time, menopause itself hasn't changed, but the lives of women certainly have. At the turn of the 20th Century, the lifespan of the average woman was 48, meaning many women never even made it to menopause. By contrast, today's women can expect to live well into their late 70s, a statistic that puts millions of women into what's known as the "post-menopausal years." The average woman, in fact, will spend one-third of her life beyond menopause, no longer concerned with a monthly menstrual period or pregnancy, but now facing some of the health challenges that come with aging and maturity.

Over the last several decades, women have been faced with a

growing amount of conflicting information about menopause, and perhaps no other health issue has generated such frenzied recommendations and opinions about the appropriate ways of thinking about, managing and "treating" menopause. As a result, many women are confused about what to "do" about menopause. For many women, minor symptoms associated with menopause can be easily managed with lifestyle changes and over-the-counter products, and for some, there's nothing but smooth sailing through "the change." For others, menopause may be a time for dialogue with their doctor.

WHAT IS MENOPAUSE?

Strictly defined, menopause is the time in a woman's life when menstruation ends and the ovaries and reproductive organs/glands begin reducing the amount of estrogen and other hormones they produced during a woman's child-bearing years.

For most women, the average age of the last menstrual period is 51, although menopause itself can begin as early as the 30s and last beyond the age of 51.

The years leading up to menopause are called perimenopause, or premenopause, and they can be brief – a few months, perhaps – or last for years. Some women begin experiencing menopause-like symptoms – hot flashes, night sweats, irregular periods, mood swings – in their mid-to-late 30s, while others never notice any symptoms at all. A woman is considered to be "postmenopausal" when she's gone a full year without a menstrual period.

The loss of estrogen means a woman's health and appearance can undergo profound changes. As estrogen wanes, the risk of heart disease increases (See Chapter 9), as does the risk of the bone-thinning disease called "osteoporosis" (See Chapter 11), and urinary tract changes that can lead to incontinence or cause more frequent urinary tract infections. For some women, the hair-graying process speeds up, and they might notice that their skin is no longer as supple as it once was. But for most women, paying attention to the important issues of exercise, diet, mental activity and personal-care means they can meet these challenges head on.

What women need to understand is that menopause is totally natural. It's a stage of life, a transition from one phase to another. It is NOT an illness that needs to be treated or fixed. Today's women have far more information and knowledge about their bodies and what to expect of the menopausal years. The good news is that some very self-directed decisions can make profound differences in how women experience this new phase of life and health.

Symptoms

Common symptoms of menopause include:

Irregular periods: Your menstrual periods may come more frequently (every two weeks) than usual or become farther apart (every few months). The flow can be light or heavy, with some women reporting heavy "gushing" or "flooding" on certain days of the period.

Hot flashes: One of the most common symptoms of menopause, so-called "hot flashes," affects about 75%-80% of menopausal women. Doctors call them a "vasomotor" symptom, meaning they affect the nerves and blood vessels, causing blood to rush through the body or to be restricted more than usual. Hot flashes can be mild or intense, and they feel like a sudden rush of heat that spreads from the chest outward to the head, neck, arms and even legs. Some women talk of a need to rip their clothes off or open a freezer door and stand in the cool air that rushes out. (Once you've had one, you'll know what it is!) Sometimes, hot flashes are accompanied by flushing and red blotching of the face, neck and body. Some women report other symptoms: nausea, headaches, dizziness and rapid heart rate. These can happen any time, but women typically report that they occur more frequently at night.

Night sweats: Have you ever woken in the middle of the night with your pajamas and linens soaking wet? That's a night sweat, a hot flash that's accompanied by severe sweating and sleeplessness.

MENOPAUSE: Bring on the Change

Emotional changes: Some women report increased irritability or moodiness, including nervousness or mild depression, as they move through menopause.

Vaginal dryness: As estrogen levels in the body wane, the functions that estrogen support begin to wane as well, and one of the jobs of estrogen is to keep tissue healthy and elastic. Some women experience vaginal dryness with menopause as the vagina walls become thinner and less elastic. Sometimes bleeding may occur, or women might feel pain or discomfort during sexual activity.

Sexual desire: Freed of the fear of pregnancy, some women find menopause sexually freeing. For other women, the symptoms and changes that accompany menopause may actually decrease sexual desire, either for emotional or hormonal reasons.

Urinary problems: The decline of hormones, that once kept the bladder elastic and firm, results in the bladder becoming less supple and prone to changes. It may not empty completely during urination, causing a constant sensation of having to "go." The chance of urinary tract infections increases, and some women may experience urinary incontinence, or the leaking of small amounts of urine out of the bladder.

Self-help approaches to menopausal symptoms

Many of the symptoms related to menopause can be handled with simple lifestyle changes or habit shifts. Some suggestions:

- Dress in layered clothing to quickly remove pieces as needed for hot flashes.
- Keep the thermostat at work and home set at a cool, comfortable level.
- Wear fabrics that "breathe" and allow for air circulation (remember, sweating helps cool the skin).
- Have cool drinks handy.
- Keep a portable fan handy.
- Exercise regularly, both to combat hot flashes and to sleep better at night.

⊛ Avoid some of the triggers that can set off hot flashes or intensify them: caffeine, alcohol, stress, extreme heat, clothes that are tight around the chest, neck or wrists and enclosed spaces.

⊛ Take measures at night to deal with hot flashes or night sweats, including using light blankets or sheets, keeping legs and feet uncovered, placing a cool washcloth on your neck or face, getting up and walking around, or taking a cool shower. If you're wide awake, why not read a good book or write a letter to make use of the time?

⊛ Use a water-soluble lubricant during sex to avoid dryness and discomfort (avoid petroleum-based lubricants because they can harbor bacteria that spread vaginal infections and they can erode the latex in condoms). If sex becomes difficult, consult your doctor or a sex therapist, because sexual activity can certainly continue well into the later years of life. Vaginal creams containing estrogen also are available for vaginal dryness.

HRT – CONTINUING CONTROVERSY

Hormone replacement therapy, once touted as a potential "cure" for large numbers of post-menopausal women, has recently generated controversy. In August 2002, part of the federally funded Women's Health Initiative was halted when researchers found that one of the major HRT drugs actually increased the risks of heart attacks and invasive breast cancer. Even though the drug had never been approved for heart disease prevention, many doctors prescribed it for that reason. Until that time, the drugs also had been used as a solution for a variety of other symptoms, including memory loss, aging skin, osteoporosis prevention and more.

The FDA urges women to talk to their doctors first about the risks and benefits of hormone replacement therapy. Just as hormone replacement therapy was never right for all women, it is not now wrong for all women. Along with their doctor's advice, some women are choosing to use HRT for temporary relief of menopausal symptoms.

Are there alternatives? Yes. Talk to your doctor about topical

MENOPAUSE: Bring on the Change

vaginal products for vaginal dryness and atrophy. Women with osteoporosis may consider non-estrogen treatments as a first option. Of course, there are other forms and formulations of estrogen and progesterone – injections, vaginal rings, skin patches and the like. This is a perfect opportunity for dialogue with your doctor. Take the time to discuss your health history and personal risk factors. Together, you should choose the best options for you.

Because some cancers may be affected by exposure to HRT, and because of its risk factors, certain women may be advised to NOT take hormone replacement therapy. They include:

❁ Those who smoke.

❁ Women who've had a breast cancer or have a family history of it.

❁ Women who are pregnant or suspect they might be.

❁ Women who have unexplained uterine bleeding.

❁ Women who have a history of blood-clotting disorders.

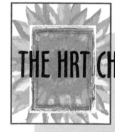

THE HRT CHOICE...and serious considerations

I f you do decide on HRT with your doctor, the FDA recommends these considerations:

❁ Take the drug "at the lowest possible dose and for the shortest period of time." For some women, that means a few months may be all that's necessary to bridge the gap from premenopause to true menopause.

❁ Be sure to undergo a yearly breast exam by a health care provider, perform monthly breast self-exams and receive a periodic mammogram, based on your age and risk factors. Most advise a yearly mammogram after age 40.

❁ Talk to your doctor about other ways to reduce risk factors for heart disease and osteoporosis.

56

PURSUING ALTERNATIVES

Rebecca Bechhold, M.D., a Cincinnati cancer specialist who treats many women with breast cancer, often is asked by her patients about HRT, and she recommends caution.

"Look at alternatives," she suggests. "There may not be great studies on things like black cohosh, evening primrose oil, flaxseed, Vitamin E and natural progesterone creams, and the information that's out there may be anecdotal, but each woman's experience is different, and some women have great success with no need for other treatments.

"Some of my patients buy a small bottle of black cohosh or evening primrose oil, for example, and try it. It's not a big investment, and if it works for you, great."

What are some herbal or natural alternatives?

Here are some ideas suggested by the Physicians Committee for Responsible Medicine and by Dr. Andrew Weil, author and integrative medicine specialist at the University of Arizona.

- A low-fat, vegetarian diet may help relieve hot flashes in some women.

- Regular exercise, such as a vigorous walk every day or other physical activity that gets the heart and lungs pumping, has overall health benefits. Many women find it relieves hot flashes and aids in better nighttime sleep during menopause.

- Black cohosh is an herb that seems to work by supporting and maintaining key female hormones, but it is not to be taken if a woman is experiencing heavy bleeding.

- Dong quai, another herb thought to support necessary female hormones, may also help some women as they move through menopause. Like black cohosh, it should not be taken if a woman is experiencing heavy bleeding.

- Vitamin E, in doses of 800 IU (international units) daily, may help with hot flashes and breast tenderness and/or lumpiness.

MENOPAUSE: Bring on the Change

* B Vitamins, a group of water-soluble vitamins, may help some women deal with the stress of menopausal symptoms.

* Evening primrose oil is a source of GLA, or gamma linolenic acid, which may help support hormone levels and may help the body use prostaglandins, which are substances that regulate tissue and muscle health.

* Soy products, more available than ever as soy milk, roasted soy nuts and soy supplements, can be natural sources of estrogen and may help maintain hormones and relieve common symptoms, including hot flashes.

Some of the symptoms associated with "low estrogen" are actually related to low progesterone, and natural progesterone creams made from soy products may alleviate hot flashes, night sweats, breast tenderness and irregular periods. Some progesterone creams are made from soy products, some from Mexican yams, and some can be compounded at pharmacies specifically for each woman. They're rubbed into the inner thigh, inner arms, neck and other soft spots on the body to be absorbed into the blood stream.

IMPROVING URINARY SYMPTOMS

If menopause brings about embarrassing or difficult symptoms with urination, several factors may be at work, and many treatment alternatives are available. Normally, the bladder is a walnut-sized organ that expands like a balloon as it fills with urine shuttled there by the kidney. A muscular tube called the urethra funnels urine out of the body during urination. Normally, the bladder and urethral muscles are firm, holding everything inside until the act of urination. When you urinate, muscles around the urethra relax, the bladder squeezes and urine streams out of the body. Then everything tightens up again until the next time.

The natural stretching of muscles that comes with aging and childbirth, along with the tissue changes associated with menopause, can lead to several problems. These include a higher risk of urinary tract infections, usually caused by bacteria that linger in the bladder, and by incontinence, the

58

leakage of small amounts of urine out of the body.

Urinary tract infections (UTIs). Usually caused by bacteria, these common infections occur far more frequently in women than in men. Other factors that lead to UTIs include frequent sexual intercourse (sometimes called "Honeymoonitis"), as well as some antibiotics, which kill "good" bacteria along with "bad" bacteria and may cause an overgrowth of infection-causing bacteria in the vagina, bladder, and even the kidneys. Symptoms of a UTI include a frequent need to urinate, a painful or burning sensation while urinating and pain that may spread to the lower back. Urine is usually cloudy and may be tinged with blood. Drink plenty of fluids, especially water, to increase urination and keep the bladder flushed out. Urinate before and after sexual intercourse, and keep the genital and anal areas clean. An estrogen-containing cream might help, too.

Urinary incontinence

Women are subject to several types of incontinence, and they include:

Urge incontinence, the most common type, means the bladder muscles are overactive and may release urine involuntarily – usually when you least expect it. You might feel a sudden need to "go" and urine may dribble out quickly, even as you're making a dash to the bathroom.

The Urinary Tract

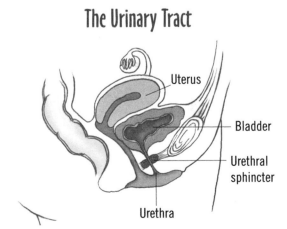

MENOPAUSE: Bring on the Change

Stress incontinence occurs when the pressure on the bladder is stronger than the urethra's ability to keep urine held back, and you may feel a sudden urge to void when doing activities that squeeze the bladder even further. Urine may leak out during laughing, coughing, sneezing or physical activity such as horseback riding or running.

Overflow incontinence occurs when the bladder doesn't empty completely during urination. Typically, small amounts of urine leak on a regular basis, and luckily, it's not as common as urge or stress incontinence.

Because urinary problems are embarrassing to women, some never seek help for a very treatable condition. But help is available for this very common – but often under-discussed – problem.

Personal-care manufacturers have created a variety of products, including absorbent pads and undergarments, which can be worn to prevent embarrassing accidents and to soak up unintentional leaks. New medications are also available to help reduce incontinence symptoms, calm overactive bladders and give women a better sense of control over their life and urinary urges. Talk to your doctor about such treatments, and be sure to ask about risks, benefits and side effects. There are surgical treatments available to repair sagging or incontinent bladders. Talk to your doctor to see which treatment is right for you. Do not assume that urinary incontinence is something to "just live with."

KEGEL EXERCISES: Shape Up!

Women can also do Kegel exercises to keep the muscles that support the bladder, urinary tract, rectum and genital area strong, firm, intact and "in shape."

Kegel exercises can be done anywhere – while you're sitting in a car at a stop light, at your desk, standing in line at the bank or cheering from the sidelines of a child's or grandchild's soccer game. And no one has to know you're doing them!

Here's how to start:

Next time you're going to the bathroom, intentionally stop and start, stop and start the flow of urine. Feel the muscles that you're using, and intentionally squeeze them for 4-5 seconds to hold urine. Then release the muscles to let urine flow freely for a short time, and squeeze again, holding it again.

Make sure that you're not tightening the abdomen, thigh or buttocks muscles. Instead, you should feel this muscular tightening especially in the area of the vagina and urethra – the so-called "pelvic floor." Once you feel the muscles that support the pelvic area, begin exercising them regularly by contracting and squeezing, holding and releasing, squeezing, holding and releasing. Repeat this 10 times in a row to make up one group of exercises. The whole process takes no more than 20 seconds. Once you get the hang of it, try to work up to 20 groups of Kegels a day.

Your doctor, a nurse or nurse practitioner can help if you don't feel that you're doing it correctly, but with time, you'll begin noticing a difference. Not only do urinary and bowel problems improve in some women, so may sexual pleasure.

Remember, no matter what happens to your body during menopause, it is another change, another phase of life that you can approach with a positive mindset and some specific ideas about staying healthy, remaining vibrant and adjusting with vigor to whatever happens next!

CHAPTER 6

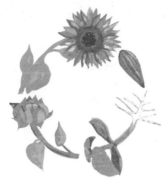

THE WOMAN'S BODY

The female body is a thing of beauty and wonder. Understanding how it works will allow you to share the joys of life as you transition through its stages. From the minute the chromosomes determine its gender at inception, the female body remains a female body for life, but is subject to constantly changing growth patterns and hormonal tides from the cradle to the grave. Hormones and DNA combine to turn quickly growing cells into uniquely female organs, tissues and functions.

And from that point on, the regular cycles of hormones regulate a woman's body. Sometimes the body functions freely and normally, sometimes it sputters and weakens. But in general, here's what happens on a normal monthly schedule once a woman reaches puberty and begins her menstrual period.

THE CYCLE

At birth, both ovaries – the tiny organs that contain all the eggs that a woman will carry through life – hold a million egg follicles, tiny balls of cells with an immature egg in the center. Starting at puberty, about 10-20 follicles start to develop each month, triggered by a hormone release in the brain called FSH – follicle-stimulating hormone. It basically tells the follicles to start "ripening" each egg by producing the hormone estrogen. Gradually, the egg moves toward the surface of the ovary for release, while estrogen already is at work telling the brain to release yet another hormone, called LH – luteinizing hormone, which causes estrogen levels to drop off. At ovulation, the egg is then released into the fallopian tubes – tiny tubes that connect the ovaries to the uterus – where it travels toward the uterus and waits to be fertilized. Released of its egg, the follicle now begins to produce another hormone – progesterone, which builds up and thickens the lining of the uterus to prepare it for pregnancy.

Sometimes, women will "feel" ovulation happen, perhaps as a twinge or cramp-like sensation in the lower abdomen or lower back.

If the egg is fertilized, it travels into the uterus and settles into the lining, where it begins drawing the necessary blood and nutrients to begin developing into a fetus.

If fertilization doesn't happen, progesterone levels eventually drop off and the bloody lining of the uterus begins to shed and release from the body, and this becomes the flow of a woman's menstrual period.

Many women fly through life with predictable, normal periods that come on a regular schedule – every 28-30 days or so. Some have irregular periods, and some suffer from what's

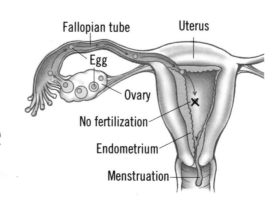

The Menstrual Cycle

called premenstrual syndrome, or PMS. Each woman's experience with PMS is different, and more than 150 different physical and emotional changes have been linked with PMS, which usually starts in the two weeks leading up to your period and stops when the period begins.

The most-common physical symptoms of PMS can usually be managed by diet, exercise, self-care and over-the-counter products. These include:

- Breast tenderness
- Bloating and weight gain of several pounds
- Abdominal cramping and gas
- Craving for sweet or salty foods
- Fatigue, sluggishness, "brain fog"
- Acne
- Headaches, including migraines
- Nausea, vomiting, diarrhea or constipation
- Back ache, joint and muscle pain
- Sleep problems

Likewise, many women notice emotional or mood changes associated with their periods, including:

- Anger and temper outbursts
- Moodiness and mood swings
- Clumsiness, klutziness and forgetfulness
- Difficulty concentrating or remembering things
- Irritability, fear and panic attacks
- Sad or depressed feelings
- Insecurity, feelings of vulnerability, unpredictable crying or "tearing up"

It's important to note that these sensations are "quite normal." It may even be important to remind our family members of this! *Those of you who frequently experience a number of these issues should look forward to menopause.*

Taking Charge

There's plenty of advice about how to "treat" or manage PMS, but each woman's body is different, each woman's symptoms are different and each woman finds solutions on her own.

Here are suggestions offered from a variety of health experts:

Exercise at least 30 minutes a day. Get enough physical activity to raise your heart rate. Try a fast walk, mild jog, bicycling, a sport you like, a lunchtime walk at a fast pace or an aerobics class. Exercise releases its own "feel-good" hormones into the body to energize you, boost your mood and relax tight tissue.

Watch what you eat. Pay attention to foods or beverages that make your PMS symptoms worse. Some women find they can prevent PMS or lessen its symptoms by avoiding alcohol, caffeine, salty foods, sweets (cookies, candy, chocolate) and replacing their sweet craving with fresh fruits. Soy foods, such as tofu and soy milk, help even out estrogen levels in some women because they contain natural plant estrogens.

Manage stress. If you know you're likely to fly off the handle or be irritable when you're suffering from PMS, take care of yourself during that time and plan your life accordingly. Try meditation, yoga, deep breathing exercises and other relaxation techniques to calm yourself down and re-establish some sense of harmony in the body. Avoid high-stress activities and ask for support and understanding from the people around you.

Control the pain. Mild over-the-counter pain relievers can often help with the minor aches, pains and headaches of PMS, but be sure to read and follow directions. Consider exercise, massage or a disposable heat wrap on the stomach for cramps.

Try a calcium-magnesium supplement (1,000 mg of each) for painful cramps. Both minerals regulate muscle tone and contractions.

Several herbs have been recommended for PMS symptoms, including evening primrose oil, black currant oil, dong quai, chaste tree or raspberry leaf tea. Talk to your pharmacist or doctor for information and advice.

Keep a positive attitude. It's often easy for people to poke fun at PMS or make jokes about it, but remember: the "joys" of being a woman are a natural part of who you are, and the changes that your body undergoes each month are nature's way of caring for the female body and the various roles it plays. Be positive about your health, and decide consciously to care for yourself in the best possible ways.

BREAST HEALTH

Funny thing about our breasts...We obsess about them from the minute they begin sprouting outward during the awkward years of puberty and spend the rest of our lives supporting them in specially-designed garments.

In reality, breasts change almost daily from the moment of puberty until menopause and beyond so that taking care of your breasts is a life-long, ever changing process.

Let's look at normal breast health and the very important things you can do to maintain healthy breasts throughout your life.

Anatomically, the breast is a very functional place, full of tissue and glands, muscles and structures that perform a variety of functions.

The chest wall is a group of muscles that fan out over the ribs and across the chest to support the breast tissue.

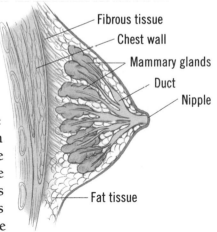

Fibrous tissue
Chest wall
Mammary glands
Duct
Nipple
Fat tissue

Fibrous tissue is what makes the breasts bulky and full. It fills in between the chest wall and the outer skin to provide support for the breast. Younger women have more fibrous tissue, which is what makes their breasts firmer. Over time, the tissue loosens as it adjusts to gravity and weight.

Fat tissue covers the breast to protect it. Each woman has a different amount of tissue in her breasts. After menopause, fat replaces the mammary glands and breasts begin to lose their firmness.

Mammary glands are tiny sacs within the breast that produce milk when a woman is breastfeeding a baby. Each breast has up to a dozen mammary glands that fill with milk and empty it through tiny ducts that travel to the nipples.

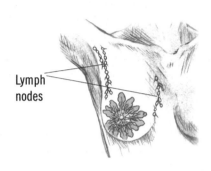

Lymph nodes are tiny bean-shaped structures that are located under the arm and beneath the breast to filter and drain lymph fluids that bathe the body. (If you've ever felt under an ill child's jaw for "swollen glands," those are lymph nodes, and they're scattered and connected throughout the body by tiny microscopic channels known as the lymphatic system). Lymph nodes are important because they tend to be the first areas to which cancerous cells in the breast can spread in women with breast cancer.

Breast Self-Exam

One of the most important things you can do to monitor the health of your breasts is a monthly breast self-exam. Scientifically, they may not be the best "tests" for finding suspicious lumps or signs of breast disease, but getting familiar with your own breasts is important in case something ever does go wrong.

In fact, Rebecca Bechhold, M.D., a Cincinnati cancer specialist, thinks women and health professionals often put too much emphasis on the correct method for performing a breast self-exam when the whole point is familiarity or "body awareness."

"Doing a breast self-exam doesn't always have to be as rigid or regimented as instructions make it out to be," Bechhold says. "Most women will come in and say, 'I was drying off after my shower and I found this lump,' and that's a very common occurrence. Whether it's your breast or your skin that changes – it's a matter of being body aware and paying attention to what's normal with your own body and your breasts so you'll know when something changes or isn't normal."

Most lumps found in the breast are not cancerous. They can be tiny calcium deposits or lumps of tissue. Some women, as part of monthly PMS symptoms, develop what doctors call "fibrocystic" conditions, or areas of lumpy hard tissue throughout the breast. Sometimes the fibrocystic areas fade as hormone levels fluctuate, and some breasts are just normally lumpy. The key is to find out what's normal in YOUR body so that you'll know when something changes. That way, you become the "expert" for your own body.

At the end of your period, spend several minutes examining your breasts for lumps, changes, dimples, scaly skin, sores, swelling, distortion – anything different that wasn't there before. It's best to do it in the shower with soapy hands, so that you can feel things better. Or lie down on the bed and gently move your fingertips in a grid pattern or circular motion in and around each breast.

The more you do it, the more you'll know what your normal breast tissue feels like and how it changes with each menstrual cycle. That way, when there are substantial changes, you'll know what's different and where.

The best time to do a breast exam depends on your age. If you're still menstruating, try to check your breasts the same time each month, preferably a few days after the end of your period when your breasts tend to be a little less lumpy and sore. If you're postmenopausal, pick the same day each month and try to check your breasts regularly.

My Personal Breast Exam Record

Age & Year	Month of Breast Self-Exam	Mammogram Date	Physical Exam Date
	— — — — — —		
———	— — — — — —	———	———

Look and Feel for Changes

Remember, you will be looking and feeling for changes in your breasts during every breast self-exam. When you have done the exam a few times, you will become familiar with the contour of your breasts, and it will be easier to discover a problem.

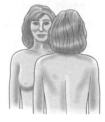

At The Mirror (with good light)
- First, relax, sitting or standing, whichever is comfortable.
- With your arms at your sides, look for changes in your breasts - lumps, thickenings, dimples or skin changes.
- Next, raise your arms above or behind your head, again looking for the same changes.

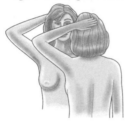

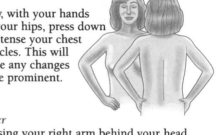

- Now, with your hands on your hips, press down and tense your chest muscles. This will make any changes more prominent.

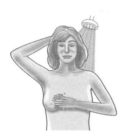

In The Shower
- Start by raising your right arm behind your head.
- With your left hand soaped, fingers held flat together, roll and press the breast firmly against the chest wall.
- Using one of the 3 motions shown below, feel a small portion of the breast at a time, until the entire breast and underarm area have been checked.
- Now repeat, raising your left arm and checking your left breast with your right hand.

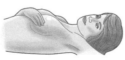

Circular   Vertical   Wedge

Lying Down
- Lie down on your back and get comfortable.
- Then, place a pillow under your right shoulder.
- Now simply repeat the process you went through in the shower, examining your right breast with your left hand.
- Move the pillow under your left shoulder and examine your left breast with your right hand. *Don't forget! If you find a problem, phone your health care provider right away.*

Getting a mammogram

Doctors now recommend a mammogram – or low-dose X-ray of the breast – as one way of identifying cancers in the breast early, when they're easier to remove and treat. Most doctors agree that mammograms are a first line of defense against breast cancer.

There are two types of mammograms. One is a screening mammogram, performed to look for abnormalities or changes related to cancer. If doctors find something unusual or suspicious on a screening mammogram, a woman is usually asked to return for a diagnostic mammogram, which is a more detailed look at the breast to hone in specifically on the changes noticed earlier. Keep in mind, too, between 10% and 20% of cancers will not be detected by an X-ray, which is why it's so important to continue performing monthly breast self-exam and schedule a yearly clinical breast exam by your doctor or a professional health care provider.

Keep these things in mind before getting a mammogram:

- Don't put on deodorant (it contains aluminum), creams or powders on the day of your mammogram. They can cloud the image.
- Schedule your appointment 1-2 weeks after your menstrual period.
- Point out any lumps or changes in your breast before the technician performs the mammogram.

The mammogram schedule

Who should get a mammogram and when?

The American Cancer Society recommends this schedule for mammograms:

- Women ages 20-30 should have a clinical breast exam by a health professional (doctor, trained nurse, etc.) every three years and should examine their own breasts every month.
- Women 40 and older should have a mammogram every year, a clinical breast exam by a health professional every

year and perform a monthly breast self-exam. Some doctors say women can have mammograms every other year from ages 40-50, but yearly mammograms are recommended after 50, because the incidence of breast cancer increases as women get older.

❀ If there's a history of breast cancer in your family, talk to your doctor about the possible need for mammograms earlier in your life.

Many women complain that mammograms hurt – so much so that some vow never to get one again. Mammograms can be uncomfortable, but talk to the technician during your mammogram if things don't feel right or are unpleasant. Relax and remind yourself that it's momentary discomfort that can prevent something even more serious if it catches breast cancer early enough to be treated successfully. It's a worthwhile trade-off!

UTERINE AND CERVICAL HEALTH

The uterus is also called the womb – the pear-shaped organ that's so stretchy and muscular it can grow to accommodate and nurture a growing fetus until birth.

That's when the uterus really does its job – during pregnancy and childbirth, but a woman's uterus requires regular checkups to monitor for other conditions or diseases, especially uterine or cervical cancer. The cervix is the muscle at the opening of the uterus into the vagina.

Every woman, once she reaches 18 or becomes sexually active, is encouraged to have a Pap smear once a year to check for signs of cancer in the cervix. During a Pap smear, a small spatula or brush is swabbed across the cervix to catch cells. Those cells are then placed on a microscopic slide and examined for any signs of changes, irregularity or abnormal growth. Talk to your doctor about follow-up treatment and a regular schedule for further Pap tests in the future.

THE WOMAN'S BODY

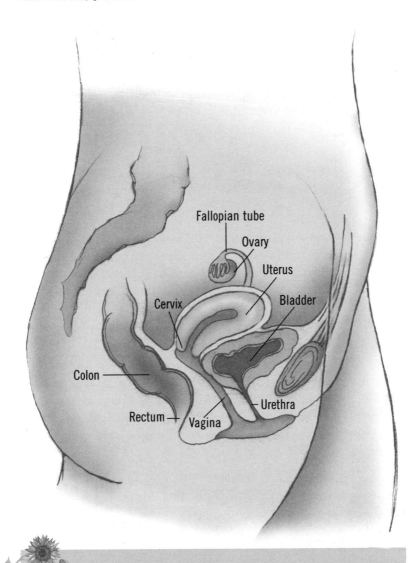

Fallopian tube
Ovary
Uterus
Cervix
Bladder
Colon
Urethra
Rectum
Vagina

Check with your doctor about some new guidelines which are being considered by The American Cancer Society regarding the frequency of Pap tests.

Where Fibroids Occur

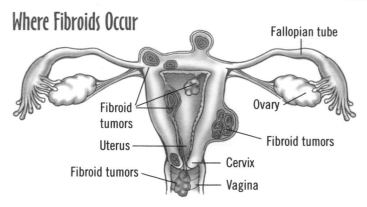

Fallopian tube

Fibroid tumors

Ovary

Fibroid tumors

Uterus

Cervix

Fibroid tumors

Vagina

Fibroids

One of the most common conditions to affect the uterus is the appearance of fibroids. They're abnormal growths, usually made of muscle and fiber tissue, that attach and grow on the walls of the uterus. About 50% of all women have fibroids at some time, and they're more common in African-American women. Fibroids can be as small as a pea or grow as large as a grapefruit.

The larger they are, the more problems they tend to create – irregular periods, heavy bleeding, pain and discomfort. Treatment may vary, from monitoring, to medication, to minimally-invasive procedures to shrink the fibroids. In severe cases, doctors may perform a hysterectomy – surgical removal of the uterus.

Endometriosis

Endometriosis is a condition that develops when the endometrium – the lining of the uterus – develops outside of the uterus and in a woman's abdominal and pelvic cavity. Sometimes tissue is found clinging to various organs and muscles in and around the abdomen, and if a woman is pre-menopausal, the tissue still responds by swelling and shrinking monthly when exposed to different hormones. Women with endometriosis usually have abdominal pain or cramping, especially right before and right after their periods, and their periods may become irregular or very heavy. Pain while urinating or during sexual intercourse is also a possible symptom. Doctors can treat endometriosis with drugs that may shrink the tissue or stop menstruation for several months. In severe cases, doctors may recommend a hysterectomy.

Hysterectomy

A hysterectomy is the surgical removal of the uterus, and may involve the ovaries as well.

Doctors may recommend a hysterectomy for a variety of reasons, including:

* Cancer of the uterus
* Fibroids that don't respond to other kinds of treatments
* Endometriosis that doesn't respond to other treatments
* Uncontrollable and heavy menstrual bleeding

You and your doctors should consider all treatment alternatives before choosing hysterectomy. These treatments may include medicines, hormones, non-invasive and/or outpatient surgical procedures and devices.

If the ovaries are healthy, there is no reason to remove them at the same time the uterus is removed, although some doctors routinely do remove them. Make sure you examine all your options, and consider at least one other opinion before deciding to have a hysterectomy.

VAGINAL HEALTH

The vagina is the muscular organ that connects the uterus with the outside of the body. It's the channel through which menstrual blood flows during a woman's period. It's also the birth canal through which a baby travels out of the uterus into the world during childbirth.

Normally, the vagina is a moist place that produces its own secretions and mucous, and harbors many bacteria to keep other germs (yeast, fungi, etc.) from growing out of proportion.

Once in a while, the normal balance of fluids and bacteria in the vagina is affected, causing an infection due to yeast or other organisms. Women may experience an abnormal discharge and frequent urination.

Most vaginal infections can be treated with over-the-counter creams that are inserted directly into the vagina, but if you've never had an infection before, see a doctor first to find out what's causing the infection. Most over-the-counter products can treat yeast infections, but different drugs may be necessary if other organisms are causing the infection. Talk to your doctor about newer, effective prescription treatments.

Women can lower their risk of getting a vaginal infection by following some simple guidelines:

- Always wear underwear that has a cotton crotch that absorbs moisture, keeping the vaginal area as dry as possible.

- Avoid wearing slacks and pants that are extremely tight in the crotch and thighs.

- Keep the genital and pubic area clean, especially before and after sexual intercourse. Never have sexual relations while you have an active infection.

- Limit your consumption of coffee, alcohol and sugar.

- Yeast infections may also be countered by reducing the amount of sugar in your diet, especially refined carbohydrates (breads, cakes, pastries, cookies, etc.) because the sugar can encourage the growth of yeast.

- Certain medicines may upset the normal bacterial balance in the body, making you more susceptible to vaginal infections. Talk to your doctor or pharmacist.

OVARIAN HEALTH

Located on each side of the uterus, and connected to it by tiny fallopian tubes, the ovaries are the organs in the body that produce eggs every month as part of a woman's reproductive cycle. In fact, when you're born, your ovaries already contain all the eggs they will carry for the rest of your life.

One of the most common problems with ovaries is ovarian cysts. They develop when the egg tissue grows and fills with fluid or blood. Normally so tiny that they are difficult to see with the naked eye, these cellular cysts can grow to 5 centimeters in diameter and cause discomfort in the stomach, pain during sexual intercourse, irregular periods, heavy bleeding and postmenopausal bleeding. There are several kinds of cysts, depending on which types of tissue are involved.

If you have a cyst, it's possible you won't have any symptoms and it will disappear on its own. Sometimes, doctors find cysts while doing a pelvic examination, and if it is causing no symptoms, they'll monitor it until it dissolves and disappears on its own. Large or persistent cysts can be drained or removed surgically, especially if doctors think they might be cancerous.

Healthy blood

One of the elements that makes blood red and rich is iron. Women are far more likely than men to not have enough red blood cells or hemoglobin – the molecules that carry oxygen – because they lose blood monthly during their menstrual periods. During pregnancy, iron loss is even more pronounced. Severe iron loss is called anemia.

Anemia causes vague symptoms, including chronic fatigue, irritability, dizziness, memory problems, shortness of breath, headaches and bone pain. Some women who are anemic look pale or ashen.

Preventing anemia is best accomplished by eating iron-rich foods. They include:

- Lean meat and liver
- Leafy greens
- Dried fruit, peas, beans
- Egg yolks
- Blackstrap molasses
- Wheat germ, whole grain breads and cereals
- Oysters

If you need extra iron, your doctor or pharmacist can recommend a supplement.

Regular checkups

Every major purchase in your life – from a new car to a water heater, a dishwasher to a curling iron – comes with a handy maintenance manual and recommended schedule of checkups and tune-ups. Unfortunately, the human body comes into the world without such a manual.

But doctors agree that a certain schedule of checkups and exams is helpful for monitoring your health, catching early signs of disease and being able to intervene quickly when your health changes.

AGE APPROPRIATE PREVENTIVE CARE TABLE

Health Activity	12-17 Years	18-24 Years	25-39 Years
Height, Weight & General Physical	annually	annually	annually
Blood Pressure/ Pulse	every other year	every other year	annually
Blood Sugar Evaluation	usually not necessary	usually not necessary	baseline, every 5 years thereafter
Immunizations	up to date with rubella titer	up to date with rubella titer	tetanus booster every 10 years
Breast Exam by Health Care Provider	teach self breast exam technique	annually*	annually*
Mammography	usually not necessary	usually not necessary	baseline before age 40
Pelvic Exam and Pap Smear	annually if sexually active	annually*	annually*
Hematocrit or Hemoglobin	every other year	every other year, chronic dieters more frequently	every other year
Cholesterol/ Triglycerides	usually not necessary	baseline age 20 and every 5 years following	5 years
Urinalysis	baseline	every 5 years	every 5 years
Thyroid	usually not necessary	usually not necessary	usually not necessary
EKG	usually not necessary	usually not necessary	usually not necessary
Stool for Occult Blood	usually not necessary	usually not necessary	usually not necessary
Bone Density	usually not necessary	usually not necessary	usually not necessary
Dental Exam	twice a year	twice a year	twice a year
Eye Exam	consult health care provider	consult health care provider	baseline exam before age 39
HIV	per risk	per risk	per risk
Skin	every two years	every two years	every year
Flexible Sigmoidoscopy	usually not necessary	usually not necessary	usually not necessary
Colonoscopy	usually not necessary	usually not necessary	usually not necessary

As recommended by the American Cancer Society * As recommended by the American College of Obstetricians
As recommended by the Academy of Ophthalmology

40-59 Years	60 and Over	Comments
annually	annually	
annually	annually	more often if a woman is on birth control pills or has a history of high blood pressure
baseline, every 5 years thereafter	every other year	
tetanus booster every 10 years	influenza vaccine yrly, pneumonia vaccine every 5 years	
annually*	annually*	breast self-exam performed monthly•
annually	annually	recommendations on mammogram may change
annually, if woman not at high risk*	annually, if woman not at high risk*	check with physician for exam timetable for post-menopausal women
every 5 years	every 3 years	nutritional anemia is common for women who menstruate, uncommon after menopause
5 years	5 years	per health care providers discretion
every year after 55	every year after 55	more often during pregnancy or in women at high risk for diabetes or renal disease
every 5 years	every 5 years	
baseline	3-5 years	more often if a woman is at high risk for heart disease
starting at age 50 and annually	annually	
starting at age 50 or if not on HRT	as doctor advises, if post-menopausal	if at risk, as recommended by health care provider
twice a year	twice a year	
every 2-4 years ♣	every 1-2 years if 65 or older ♣	more frequent visits if experiencing vision problems
per risk	per risk	
every year	every year	more frequently if needed
at age 50 and every five years after	every 5 years	frequency depends on risk
at age 50 and every ten years after	every 10 years	if at risk, as recommended by health care provider

The above screenings are guidelines only. If you are experiencing any signs or symptoms that are worrisome to you, talk to your health care provider and ask about having a particular screening done.

CHAPTER 7

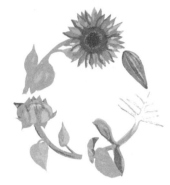

GOOD STRESS, BAD STRESS

Mention the word "stress" to just about any woman today, and she'll rattle off a list of stressful "stuff" in her life – job, health, kids, worries, bills, aging parents, an old car, a new house...the list can be endless!

But, in reality, stress is a good-bad phenomenon.

There's good stress – the kind of stress that, in our primitive lives, sent a shot of adrenaline and other hormones through our system so we could dart out of the way of oncoming danger or save ourselves in times of crisis.

Author Hans Seyle is credited with describing "stress" in its modern usage, and he often described "good stress" as the bodily reaction that took place every time a primitive human instinctually produced the "fight or flight" instinct to run away, for example, from a sabre-tooth tiger.

But there's negative stress, too – and it's stress that wears women down over time, depleting bodies of energy, sapping reserves, overworking vital organs and making the body less well equipped to protect itself from disease and infection.

Over time, the same hormones and chemicals that supercharge the body for "fight or flight" can have a negative effect, pushing it into a constant state of alertness that can cause chronic problems, ranging from pain to heart disease, skin problems to irritable bowels, high blood pressure to tension headaches.

THE STRESS REACTION

But here's what's most important about stress – it can make you sick.

How you react to stress – good or bad – will determine whether you succumb to its negative influences or whether you learn how to survive it and lessen its impact on your health, your mental state and your outlook on life.

That's right. Most of what we think of today as negative stress is rooted in our coping abilities – the mindsets, thought patterns, physical behaviors and habits that we develop and learn to deal with when a stress stimulus presents itself.

So let's look at what stress is, and what you can do to get a grip, literally and figuratively.

What is stress?

The non-profit American Stress Institute defines stress in several ways.

There's **external stress** – factors outside the body that have an impact on it, such as pain, heat, cold, danger, poor working conditions, abusive relationships, constant loud noises and the like.

And there's **internal stress**, which can be physical (infections, hunger, swelling, tumors) or psychological, such as intense worry, fear or loneliness.

Ideally, stress should be short-term. It should be something that you learn to deal with, and then it goes away. If the room becomes too hot, open a window and the heat dissipates – taking the stress of the heat with it. If poor working conditions wear you down on the job, talk with a supervisor and work toward an improvement plan.

Chronic stress, though, occurs when short-term solutions simply aren't available or don't work, so you continue to feel and react to the negative stress.

And stress reactions create a chemical-soup mixture in your body that can produce a variety of symptoms, feelings and changes.

The American Stress Institute notes that women in general are at higher risk than men for stress-related health problems, that minority women have higher levels of stress than the general female population, and that working mothers, in particular, face some of the highest stress levels among any group.

What stress does inside your body

When your body's under stress, it gets busy – too busy for its own good. Let's take a look at what happens in the body.

- Any kind of stress releases steroid hormones into the body. These hormones marshal your heart, lungs, circulation, metabolism, immune system and skin to be prepared for an immediate reaction.

- The heart rate and breathing speed up, blood is pooled away from the limbs toward your heart for better efficiency, skin sweats and becomes clammy to keep the body from overheating, white blood cells are sent to the body's front lines in case of injury, and your body's ability to digest food shuts down temporarily because it wants you to focus on removing yourself from danger.

- Chemical messengers called neurotransmitters flood the body, triggering feelings and reactions. You may sense fear. Your vision and hearing will be more alert. Your memory may be affected because the body wants you to react quickly, not intellectually.

But if the stress doesn't go away immediately, your body stays in a constant state of readiness, continually pumping out hormones and chemicals intended to keep you on edge. Over time, your organs, tissues, nerves, blood cells and entire systems can begin to wear out from being over-stimulated, and as they begin to malfunction, they become imbalanced and out of whack.

In short, stress can make you sick.

What Chronic Stress Can Do Inside Your Body

Stress itself is often thought of as an entity that's hard to pin down. It's something out there, not truly definable, usually caused by something else.

But research shows that stress can create very physical symptoms, if it's left unanswered or unheeded. Among them:

- High blood pressure
- Headaches/migraines
- Strokes
- Heart attacks
- Ulcers
- Susceptibility to the common cold, infections and allergies
- Memory problems
- Shortness of breath
- Racing/pounding heart beat
- Inability to relax
- Immune disorders (eczema, lupus, arthritis)
- Cancer
- Heartburn
- Stomach/digestion problems (irritable bowel syndrome, peptic ulcers)
- Eating problems (weight gain, weight loss, eating disorders)
- Diabetes (insulin-resistant)
- Sleep problems
- Sexual and reproductive dysfunction
- Unexplained hair loss (alopecia)
- Chronic pain

Getting A Grip

Remember, it's how you REACT to stress that determines how well you'll be able to manage the physical changes inside your body. And reacting to stress requires that you be conscious of the effect it's having on you.

Take this self-assessment to find out how busy and tightly wound your life actually is. Answer each question with a simple **"Yes"** or **"No"**.

Do it in pencil, so you can retake the assessment after you practice your stress-relieving techniques on the following pages.

1. At the end of a day, I feel frustrated because I did not accomplish all that I had planned. ❑ Yes ❑ No

2. I find myself trying to be everything to everybody. ❑ Yes ❑ No

3. My physical health is affected by stress in my life. ❑ Yes ❑ No

4. My life is a series of crises. ❑ Yes ❑ No

5. I need extra help managing my work and family responsibilities. ❑ Yes ❑ No

6. Money is a source of conflict for me. ❑ Yes ❑ No

7. I have difficulty finding time for activities with my family or partner. ❑ Yes ❑ No

8. My work usually interferes with my family life. ❑ Yes ❑ No

       TOTAL "Yes"____   TOTAL "No"____

9. The members of my family share in the care and maintenance of our home. ❑ Yes ❑ No

10. I feel that my working conditions are good. ❑ Yes ❑ No

11. My family life interferes with my work. ❑ Yes ❑ No

12. I feel successful about balancing my work and family roles. ❑ Yes ❑ No

13. I feel physically capable of meeting the day's challenges because I set aside time in my life for ME. ❑ Yes ❑ No

14. I feel I can successfully handle any obstacle ☐ **Yes** ☐ **No**
thrown my way, with the help of family, friends
and co-workers.

15. I may not have as much as I would like, but ☐ **Yes** ☐ **No**
I make ends meet by communicating with my family.

TOTAL "Yes"_____   **TOTAL "No"_____**

HOW DID YOU DO? If you answered **"No"** to more than 4
questions in section 1-8 and/or if you answered **"Yes"** to more
than 3 questions in 9-15, you are likely dealing with stress in
your life. Use this list as a resource for identifying potentially
troublesome areas, and use the rest of this chapter for finding
possible tips, solutions and coping mechanisms.

MANAGING STRESS

Here are a few time-tested techniques for relieving stress and
restoring balance in your body, recommended by the American
Stress Institute.

※**Relaxation Techniques,** such as yoga, relaxation CDs
and cassette tapes, visual imagery and quiet time, just for
you, every day. Make it a daily part of your routine.

※**Deep Breathing.** It's easy to learn, and you can use it
wherever and whenever you need it.

※**Muscle Relaxation.** Start from the top of your head and
gradually loosen and relax every muscle and joint until
you reach your toes. Feel the difference?

※**Meditation.** Cultures around the world have used
meditation for thousands of years to calm the
body and slow the breathing. Consciously focus
inward and relax the body and mind. Buy a tape
or take a class.

※**Biofeedback** is a way of training the brain and
thought patterns to relax and focus
inward. Talk to your doctor or
alternative health provider about
biofeedback.

✻**Massage therapy** is a sheer treat that can bring instantaneous relaxation and relief, physically and mentally.

✻**Keep a journal or stress diary.** Putting your thoughts on paper can help release a lot of stress in your life. Writing can help organize your thinking. Continue to go back and read previous journal entries to get a sense of where you've been and where you're going.

✻**Eat a healthy diet.** Your body requires proper balanced nutrition simply to stay as balanced as possible.

S-T-R-E-T-C-H Away Your Stress!

For thousands of years, practitioners of yoga have used their stretching techniques, deep breathing and conscious relaxation to deal with stress. Two of our expert presenters at our Speaking of Women's Health conferences are Dr. Deborah Kern (www.deborahkern.com) and Lilias Folan (www.liliasyoga.com). If you've taken their class or seen their tapes, or if you've ever tried any type of yoga, you know how relaxed and calm you can feel after a session of moving, stretching, breathing and relaxing your body. Consider the immediate stress-relief benefits that come simply from stretching your body's tissues: **enhances breathing, improves blood circulation, re-aligns and opens the spine, elongates muscles and surrounding tissues and counters the compressing effects of gravity on the body.**

Don't know where to start? Check at your local YWCA, YMCA, community center, women's group, church or fitness center. Many now offer yoga sessions on a regular basis. Or, you may wish to begin your mornings with a video-taped yoga session with one of our experts.

Beating Stress in the Mind

Part of the approach to managing how you react to stress is managing how you THINK about stress. The web site www.mindtools.com suggests these questions to ask yourself when assessing stress in your life and thinking about new ways to tackle it. **Next time a stressful situation presents itself, ask yourself these questions:**

? Is this really a problem at all?

? Is this a problem that anyone else has now, or has faced in the past? (If so, can you learn from what they've done?)

? Can you break down this seemingly huge problem into smaller, easier-to-solve problems?

? If you're facing more than one problem, can you put them in order and deal with them in a way that you don't feel so overwhelmed?

? Does it really matter? Will this issue resolve itself?

FOODS AND SUBSTANCES THAT MAY CAUSE STRESS

Plenty of factors in your life can feel stressful, but keep in mind that certain foods can make stressful reactions seem even worse. Common foods that can intensify the effects of stress include:

Caffeine. Remember, it's a stimulant. Just drinking coffee causes typical stress reactions – a pumping heart, anxiety and nervousness. Consider cutting down on coffee and soda consumption for awhile. There are plenty of alternatives available today, from herbal teas to nutrient-rich waters.

Alcohol. In small doses, alcohol can help you relax, but alcohol can also disrupt sleep and can cause long-term bodily damage to key organs and mental faculties.

Nicotine. Although it may make you FEEL relaxed, nicotine is also a stimulant. It speeds up your heart and causes a variety of other changes in the body. DO YOU NEED ANOTHER REASON TO QUIT??? (See Chapter 12)

Sugary foods. Foods that are high in sugars can play havoc with your body's insulin levels. This is a good opportunity to bring fresh fruits, nuts and multi-grain health bars into your diet.

Next time someone mentions the word stress, you may be the one suggesting the solutions!

CHAPTER 8

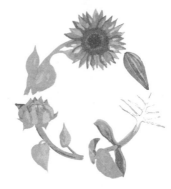

CHRONIC CONDITIONS

Making the Most of Life, Regardless of What You've Got

Some people are blessed with a healthy body, experiencing little or no chronic pain or discomfort. Some of this "luck" is simply due to their genetic makeup, but others are making their own "luck" by opting for healthful decisions. Still others do have to think about and worry about everyday activities because – for whatever reason – they have a chronic, underlying health problem or condition...one that won't go away, or is stubborn enough to require ongoing attention and treatment.

Even so, many people with chronic health conditions may sail through life, because they've adopted the proper lifestyle habits and mindsets to manage, control and live with an underlying disease with a positive attitude.

And that's the key to living with a chronic disease, whether it's asthma or diabetes, multiple sclerosis or a thyroid problem.

Women who put the emphasis on "living with" a chronic condition, and not on the condition itself, tend to have better outcomes, better health and a more positive spirit, say health experts. But, getting to that mindset requires a conscious decision and dedication, because choosing the alternative – ignorance or avoidance, negativity or apathy – may cause more problems than the chronic condition itself.

"If you do have a chronic illness, you have got to prioritize taking care of yourself so that you don't then end up with all the complications you'll have if you don't take care of yourself," says Marilyn Gaston, M.D., former Assistant Surgeon General and co-author of *Prime Time: the African-American Woman's Complete Guide to Mid-Life Health and Wellness* (Random House). "The hard part is getting women to prioritize themselves." Sometimes, as women, we have to put ourselves first, so that we feel well enough to meet all of our responsibilities.

Gaston says that a critical part of managing a chronic disease is having the proper mental attitude – learning to live fully with the disease rather than adopting the mindset that it's a heavy burden to be borne or an insurmountable challenge.

"It's an approach to life that's needed – it doesn't matter what the disease or what the issue is," she explains. "It's a matter of approaching every challenge as an opportunity." Women who have a wonderful self-concept, a wonderful belief in themselves, in the world and in life in general, are the ones who see whatever they have to deal with and react appropriately. Sometimes, they even see it as an opportunity to grow.

Critically important is having a support network on which to depend for emotional, physical and day-to-day encouragement and help, Gaston says. Women with multiple sclerosis, for example, may benefit tremendously by having a network of friends to help them with tasks they cannot tackle on their own, or by having a network of friends who also have multiple sclerosis so they can learn from each other and draw strength from each other's challenges and successes. In fact, many women today who do not have a physical network of friends, often turn to online support groups and chat rooms to connect with other women for bonding, help, advice and a "cyber-shoulder" on which to lean.

"You cannot deal with any of this stuff by yourself, and I

think that's something that we, as women, need to learn," Gaston says. "Often, we're more prone to 'bear the burden,' yet having a network and using that network is very important, whether it's a chronic illness or financial difficulty or family problems you're facing."

Let's look at some common chronic health problems and what can be done about them.

ASTHMA

According to the Asthma and Allergy Foundation of America (AAFA), only three diseases in the U.S. are experiencing increasing death rates, and one of those is asthma (the other two are AIDS and tuberculosis). Asthma is, indeed, on the rise in America, not just in adults, but in children as well. In fact, it's now the single largest reason that children miss school in America today.

There are gender and ethnic differences in asthma, too. Women are more likely to die of asthma than men, and African-Americans are three times more likely to be hospitalized for asthma and to die of asthma than Caucasians.

Pharynx
Esophagus
Bronchi
Sinuses
Larynx
Trachea
Bronchial tubes
Diaphragm

Why is asthma on the rise, and what can you do about it?

There are many possible reasons for the increase in asthma. These include:

⊛ Worsening air pollution

⊛ Exposure to indoor allergens in air-tight homes

⊛ Exposure to toxic chemicals or environmental triggers

⊛ Lack of access to adequate medical care and follow up

CHRONIC CONDITIONS

Some mind-body experts also link asthma with stress, not as a cause of the disease but as something that can cause a "suffocating" feeling or a heaviness that makes it difficult to catch one's breath or move through life freely.

Whatever the reasons and causes, asthma is one of those diseases that can be managed if those who have it seek medical care, institute the necessary lifestyle changes to avoid or prevent flare-ups, and take the necessary medicines and treatments to keep it from worsening.

During an asthma attack, the airway that connects the mouth and nose with the lungs becomes blocked or narrowed. The airways and branches of the lungs may swell, limiting the amount of air that passes in and out. Muscles can tighten and squeeze the lungs; again making breathing difficult, and sometimes mucous builds up inside the breathing passages, further blocking air's ability to move in and out freely.

The most common triggers of asthma are:

⊛ Dust mites

⊛ Mold

⊛ Pollen

⊛ Animal dander or cockroaches

⊛ Certain foods (nuts, shellfish, eggs, corn, wheat)

⊛ Tobacco smoke

⊛ Exercise, especially in cold air

⊛ Hormonal changes

Treating asthma

Every person's experience with asthma is different, and having asthma doesn't mean you have to limit your activities. In fact, many Olympic and professional athletes experience asthma, and they do just fine. The key is knowing what triggers your symptoms and trying to avoid them, keeping your body healthy to fight off asthma attacks and having the necessary medical treatments to intervene.

Typically, the drugs used to treat asthma are grouped into two types:

- Quick-relief medicines are used to control the immediate symptoms of an asthma attack. Bronchodialators, or inhalers, can be used to open the breathing passages while an attack is happening.

- Other medicines can be used long-term to keep the body's immune system under control so that it doesn't react to every potential trigger with an asthma attack. Over time, they help lessen the frequency and severity of episodes, according to AAFA.

Many asthma medicines have side effects – jitteriness, muscle twitches, fatigue and nausea. As with all drugs, talk to your doctor and pharmacist about risks, benefits and side effects.

Some people also find that relieving daily stress can lessen asthma attacks. Simple measures such as regular massages, meditation, relaxation exercises and cassette tapes can also help. This may be a perfect opportunity to try some simple, gentle yoga techniques.

Avoiding your triggers can also keep full-blown asthma attacks at bay. If it means you have to ask visitors not to smoke in your house, that's your right, and many people now have no-smoking households and work environments for health reasons.

If seasonal allergies – pollens in spring, grasses in summer, ragweed in the fall – set off asthma attacks, keep doors and windows closed during those times. Use air conditioning and make sure to take your medicines during times when you're most vulnerable.

With proper medical care, most people with asthma can manage their disease and symptoms with confidence.

ALLERGIES

Itchy eyes. Runny nose. Tickly sinuses. Rashes and hives. Anyone who's ever had an allergic reaction is more than familiar with the symptoms, and allergies are now the sixth-leading cause of chronic disease in the U.S., according to the AAFA.

Allergies occur when the body reacts inappropriately to anything that enters it – is breathed in, eaten or by contact with the skin. Maybe it's a piece of airborne dust, or a food protein or a chemical in a drug. If the body doesn't recognize that particle, it sets up an immune-system reaction, treating the invader as if it's a foreign object. Tiny cells, called mast cells, are released into the bloodstream, and they eventually trigger the release of chemicals called histamines. Histamines cause the eyes and nose to release mucous, causing the watery, sneezy, itchy symptoms common in an allergy attack. In severe cases, breathing can also become difficult.

Common Allergy Sources

INHALED ALLERGENS	CONTACT ALLERGENS	INGESTED ALLERGENS
Pollens	Plants and insect venom	Foods
Molds/fungi	Drugs	Drugs
House dust mites	Cosmetics	
Animal danders	Jewelry (e.g., nickel, silver, etc.)	
Cockroaches	Latex products	
Latex particles	Occupational chemical/dyes	

People can be allergic to many things.

While most allergies are not curable, they are certainly manageable. If you know what causes your allergic reactions, try as much as possible to avoid them. Use air conditioning in spring/summer/fall to keep airborne particles outside. If you're allergic to family pets, consider keeping them out of bedrooms and other living areas – or finding a proper home for the pet elsewhere. Use allergy-control bedding and coverings that limit dust dispersion. Talk to your pharmacist about alternative remedies – Vitamin C or other herbs/supplements that may ease the symptoms of allergic reactions. Talk to your doctor about antihistamines or other allergy-control products, many of them now long-acting. Be sure to read side effects and possible reactions. If you're severely allergic – usually to bee stings, insect bites or certain foods – talk to your doctor about having emergency kits on hand to stop life-threatening reactions until you can call 911 and get to the hospital. Usually, these are injection kits containing epinephrine, a substance that can keep the immune-system reaction at bay until you can get to the hospital for emergency treatment.

And remember, some allergic reactions can cut off breathing and turn deadly very quickly, so don't hesitate!

ARTHRITIS

If you think only older women get arthritis, think again. Although it's more common in older women, younger women can develop arthritis as well.

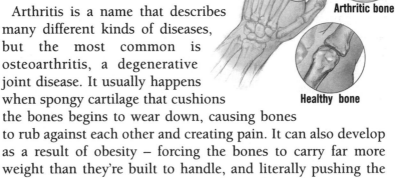

Arthritic bone

Arthritis is a name that describes many different kinds of diseases, but the most common is osteoarthritis, a degenerative joint disease. It usually happens when spongy cartilage that cushions

Healthy bone

the bones begins to wear down, causing bones to rub against each other and creating pain. It can also develop as a result of obesity – forcing the bones to carry far more weight than they're built to handle, and literally pushing the bones on top of each other in ways that make walking, moving, sleeping and activity painful or uncomfortable.

These are some of the common symptoms of arthritis that might make you want to talk to your doctor:

- Joint pain that gets worse with activity and better with rest.
- Joint stiffness that's worse in the morning but disappears in about 30 minutes.
- Stiffness in a joint after lengthy periods of inactivity.
- A "grinding" or "sandy" feeling in a joint when it's moved.
- Limited ability to move a joint freely.
- Bone swelling around an affected joint, usually a sign of rheumatoid arthritis, which is marked by chronic swelling of the joints and some internal organs.

CHRONIC CONDITIONS

Managing arthritis

Some simple lifestyle changes may sometimes help you cope with arthritis symptoms.

Most experts agree that exercise is important to keep joints moving and as fluid as possible. Many community centers and fitness centers offer exercise programs that put very little stress and strain on the joints – classes such as water aerobics or gentle yoga. Not only will they make your body feel better and more mobile, you'll get the mental boost that comes with exercise, as well.

Likewise, stretching is critical in keeping symptoms under control or even lessening them altogether. Sometimes bones rub against each other because the tissue around them is tightened and immobile from lack of use or lack of exercise. Yoga, Pilates, low-impact aerobics, walking, even lying on the floor several times a day and consciously stretching, can relieve much of this tightness, "rubbing" or "sandpapery" feeling in the joints. Remember, if you don't use it, you lose it!

Range-of-motion and strengthening exercises also can help relieve the painful sensations in the joints. These include exercises that require big sweeping movements of the arms and legs, such as low-impact aerobics, lifting hand weights, reaching, bending, yoga and Pilates.

Physical therapy can help improve flexibility and strengthen muscles. This is something to discuss with your doctor.

If needed, losing weight can go a long way to relieving and even reversing arthritis pain.

Over-the-counter topical rubs are now available to provide temporary pain relief. Some of these contain pain-relief compounds or something called capsaicin, which is the active ingredient in chili peppers. It stimulates nerve endings so that the pain of arthritis eventually lessens.

Over-the-counter pain relievers are used by many people with arthritis. These include aspirin, acetaminophen and ibuprofen. Long-term use of these drugs may cause digestive and stomach problems, so talk to your doctor or pharmacist about the best use of these kinds of medicines. Doctors also can prescribe stronger versions of these drugs, but again, discuss the risks, benefits and side effects.

The Physician Committee for Responsible Medicine (PCRM) also urges arthritis sufferers to examine their diets because of growing evidence that food allergies can trigger arthritis symptoms and joint pains. Common foods linked to arthritis include dairy products, corn, meats, grains, eggs, citrus fruits, potatoes, tomatoes, nuts and coffee. Try eliminating a certain food from your diet for a week or more, and pay attention to how your symptoms change. If they ease, remove the offending food from your diet altogether. If not, move to other foods to try to identify those that can cause arthritis-like pain.

PCRM also says two fatty acids found in plants (alpha-linolenic acid or ALA, and gamma-linolenic acid, or GLA) can have pain-relief properties for arthritis. These acids can be found in borage oil, flaxseed oil, evening primrose oil, blackcurrant oil and hemp oil. The ALA and GLA oils also can be found in vegetables, beans and peas.

Some alternative healers also recommend ginger as a natural product to reduce pain and swelling.

When exploring complementary or alternative therapies, always consult your doctor to ensure that it is appropriate for you.

Good News on the Horizon

Researchers continue to make important strides in understanding how osteoarthritis destroys cartilage and how the disease progresses. Until recently, osteoarthritis has been viewed primarily as a joint disease, and the role of poor bone health was not well understood. Today, scientists have determined that changes in the underlying structure of bone around the joint area may have a greater effect on cartilage health than previously assumed. The key to stopping the progression of osteoarthritis may lie in preserving bone structure. This has led to funding of controlled clinical studies to look at the potential value of pharmaceutical therapies, which have a positive effect on bone health.

CHRONIC CONDITIONS

DIABETES

One of the alarming trends of the last decade has been a dramatic increase in the incidence of diabetes. While some people get diabetes as children for genetic or congenital reasons, much of the growth of the disease is directly linked to the growing waistlines of the American population. **The most common form of diabetes is directly linked to obesity and weight gain, and that's why it's on the increase.**

People with diabetes have too much glucose, or a form of sugar, in the blood. Normally, the pancreas produces a chemical called insulin that converts glucose into energy for immediate use by the body or stores it as fat if the body doesn't need it. Glucose gets into the bloodstream through the food you eat.

The disease itself can affect children and adults, and it's growing in both populations. In fact, experts estimate that up to two-thirds of people who have diabetes don't know they have it and aren't being treated for it. Diabetes is also more prevalent in African-Americans, Latinos and Native Americans than Caucasians, and more common as people get older.

There are two basic types of diabetes

Type 1, or Juvenile Diabetes, usually starts in children or before age 20 and occurs when the body fails to produce insulin. It affects about 5%-10% of the population. People with Type 1 diabetes have to take daily injections of insulin because their bodies can't make it on their own.

Type 2 is the most common form of diabetes, and the one that's on the rise. It used to be called Adult-Onset Diabetes because it mostly occurred in middle-aged adults. Due to growing weight problems and obesity in children and teens, now even younger people are developing Type 2 diabetes. The body still produces insulin, but it either can't produce enough or the body does not use it well enough to convert glucose to energy. People who have "pre-diabetes" have blood glucose levels that are higher than normal but not high enough to be officially diagnosed as having Type 2 diabetes.

Symptoms

No matter what type of diabetes is involved, the symptoms are similar. They include:

- Constant thirst and hunger
- Frequent urination of large volumes of urine
- Frequent infections of the bladder, skin, vagina or urinary tract (because of excess sugar in the body)
- Blurry vision
- Occasional nausea/vomiting
- Fatigue
- Increased appetite but unexplained weight loss
- Poor wound healing

Managing diabetes

Diabetes is a disease to be concerned about, because if it's left untreated, it can cause several complications. The most common ones include kidney damage, vision loss (retinopathy), poor circulation, or damage to nerves in the body (neuropathy). The last two complications can have severe consequences. If not addressed, they may lead to digestive problems, organ failure or amputation, if blood is not adequately delivered to the extremities, especially the feet.

For those with Type I diabetes, daily injections of insulin are needed, as are the regular blood tests that must be done to monitor blood sugar levels constantly and adjust insulin doses accordingly. Some people with Type 2 diabetes may use oral medicines that help regulate blood sugar.

For many people, losing weight, managing what they eat and exercising regularly, can relieve or even reverse some of the most common problems and symptoms associated with diabetes. As part of your treatment program, you'll be advised to meet with a dietitian to find a food plan that works for you, both to manage your blood sugar levels and to help you lose weight. Eat a balanced diet and do not overeat. Some people are able to reduce or eliminate oral glucose medicines if they can lose enough weight and continue exercising to keep blood sugar levels under control.

CHRONIC CONDITIONS

Other approaches

Relieve stress. Stress can worsen diabetic symptoms, or cause chemical changes in the body that interfere with glucose reactions, so learning to manage stress is important for people with diabetes.

Don't rush your meals. Eat slowly and consciously, and choose foods that fit your diabetic diet.

Exercise can help tremendously, not only to make symptoms more manageable but also to actually prevent and reverse diabetes. According to the National Diabetes Education program, modest weight loss and regular physical activity – such as walking 30 minutes a day five days a week – can cut the risk of developing Type 2 diabetes by more than half in people who have pre-diabetic conditions. Weight loss and activity worked for people of every ethnic and racial group, and they were especially helpful in people over 65.

Lose weight. "Fat is a problem for diabetes," according to the Physicians Committee for Responsible Medicine. "The more fat there is in the diet, the harder time insulin has in getting sugar into the cell…(and) minimizing fat intake and reducing body fat help insulin do its job much better." The good news is that a weight loss of 5 to 10% can decrease blood pressure and cholesterol levels and IMPROVE HEALTH! Sound like a challenge? Consider that if you weigh 150 pounds, a 5% weight loss is less than 10 pounds! In addition, recent research now suggests that a 5 to 7% weight loss may actually prevent Type 2 Diabetes in people at high risk for the disease.

Is there a diabetic diet?

People with diabetes used to be advised to avoid sugars, and limiting sugar is still one of the recommendations, especially sugars that are "hidden" in foods such as baked goods, processed foods, soft drinks, breakfast foods and the like. But now the emphasis is on a balanced diet. The American Diabetes Association points out that "no single food will supply all the nutrients your body needs, so good nutrition means eating a variety of foods."

People with diabetes are urged to eat:

- Plenty of fruits and vegetables
- Plenty of whole grains, cereals and bread
- Dairy products
- Meat, fish, poultry, eggs, dried beans and nuts – but choose lean, low-fat products that are low in cholesterol

WHO'S AT RISK?

You're considered at risk for diabetes if you:

- Are overweight, and the greater the weight gain, the higher your risk.
- Are inactive.
- Have high blood pressure.
- Are 45 or older, although younger and younger Americans are developing diabetes from weight gain and lack of exercise.
- Have a family history of diabetes, a history of gestational diabetes (during pregnancy) or gave birth to a baby weighing more than 9 pounds.
- Belong to an ethnic or minority group, including African-American, Hispanic American/Latino, American Indian and Asian American/Pacific Islanders.

MULTIPLE SCLEROSIS

It might begin as a numb feeling in the fingers or toes. Without notice, simple things like pulling on a pair of pantyhose or writing a child's permission slip might become difficult. For many women, these seemingly minor symptoms can be the early signs of multiple sclerosis.

For reasons not fully understood, multiple sclerosis affects women almost twice as frequently as men, and for reasons that seem even stranger, it's more common in parts of the world in northern climates. In fact, the farther north of the equator you live, the higher your risk of multiple sclerosis.

CHRONIC CONDITIONS

Multiple sclerosis is so elusive, in fact, that doctors still aren't exactly sure what causes it. It's thought to be an autoimmune disorder – in which the body recognizes its own tissue as foreign and begins attacking it. In MS, the protective covering of nerve fibers is destroyed or damaged, negatively affecting the body's ability to send messages between the brain, spinal cord and the rest of the body. It can run in families, although a genetic link is not yet established. Some experts believe that people may have a genetic predisposition for multiple sclerosis – meaning the tendency to develop it is always possible but must be activated by some sort of trigger, such as an infection, exposure to something in the environment or other unknown factors.

Symptoms of MS can be mild or severe, and they can start quickly and worsen just as quickly, or start slowly and remain low-level for years and years. The disease varies widely from person to person. Some live full, productive lives with MS, while about 25% end up disabled or bedridden because of their inability to move and work normally. Common symptoms, according to the National Multiple Sclerosis Society, are:

- Weakness, tingling, numbness or impaired sensation
- Poor coordination, problems with balance
- Fatigue or weakness
- Blurred vision or involuntary rapid eye movement
- Tremors, spastic muscles or muscle stiffness
- Slurred speech
- Bladder or bowel problems
- Unstable walking
- Sexual dysfunction
- Sensitivity to heat or cold
- Mood swings, memory problems, judgment or reasoning impairment
- In severe cases, partial or complete paralysis

Multiple sclerosis is usually a disease that doctors diagnose after ruling out a variety of other possible diseases. Because MS varies so much from woman to woman, no clear diagnostic test is available, although doctors will make the decision after a variety of tests – a complete medical history, neurological exam, magnetic images of the brain (MRI), spinal tap, central-nervous-system reaction tests and intellectual function tests. It's always wise to get a second opinion, too, especially for such a difficult diagnosis.

The good news is that research is leading to a variety of treatments for MS, some which can shorten attacks of the disease, delay the onset of permanent disabilities or reduce signs of injury within the brain. The drugs currently approved for MS include forms of interferon, an immune-system substance. Another option is a synthetic drug that mimics a component of the covering of nerve fibers. Other drugs can be used on a symptom-by-symptom basis, such as muscle relaxants for muscle problems or bladder-control drugs for women with urinary problems.

Women with MS also can rely on a variety of supportive therapies to help deal with the symptoms they experience. Physical therapy can help with balance, coordination and weakness problems. Occupational therapy can help women re-learn tasks to remain as independent as possible. Speech therapy can help women who have difficulty speaking or swallowing because of muscle or nerve problems. Cognitive rehabilitation can help improve memory, attention, information processing and other thinking properties. Some women find that computers are helpful tools to communicate with other women in "cyber" support groups.

As with many diseases, exercise can improve overall health and prevent complications, but it must be tailored for each individual woman.

The MS Society recommends a positive approach to help deal with stress and depression, both of which are common reactions to a chronic disease like this.

CHRONIC CONDITIONS

® Keep as active as possible, mentally and physically.

® Manage your time to save energy for things that are most important.

® Set priorities and simplify your life, based on what you can accomplish.

® Learn relaxation or meditation exercises.

® Get help for things you can't accomplish on your own or for difficult problems.

® Make time for fun, and maintain a sense of humor.

® Set realistic goals and expectations.

® Work on accepting what you cannot change.

As with all chronic conditions, finding a doctor who is current on MS diagnosis and treatment, and whose advice and support you trust, is critical to maintaining your own health and sense of well-being. MS can have many different symptoms and components, and it's important to build a health care team who is knowledgeable and willing to help you tackle all of the challenges that you face.

FIBROMYALGIA

Fibromyalgia syndrome (FMS) is a widespread musculoskeletal pain and fatigue disorder for which the cause is still unknown. Fibromyalgia means pain in the muscles, ligaments and tendons. More women than men are affected by fibromyalgia.

Many patients with fibromyalgia describe symptoms similar to a bad flu. Every muscle in the body aches.

Symptoms may include:
® Pain

® Fatigue

® Sleep disorder

® Irritable Bowel and/or Bladder Syndrome

® Chronic headaches

® Painful menstrual periods

- Chest pain
- Morning stiffness
- Cognitive or memory impairment
- Numbness and tingling sensations, muscle twitching, dry eyes and mouth
- Impaired coordination
- **Temporomandibular Joint Dysfunction Syndrome -** This syndrome, sometimes referred to as TMJ, causes tremendous face and head pain in one quarter of FMS patients.
- **Multiple Chemical Sensitivity Syndrome** - Sensitivities to odors, noise, bright lights, medications and various foods is common in roughly 50% of FMS patients.

Aggravating factors:
- Changes in weather, cold or drafty environments
- Hormonal fluctuations (premenstrual and menopausal states)
- Stress, depression, anxiety
- Over-exertion

Common treatments:
Traditional treatments are geared toward improving the quality of sleep, as well as reducing pain. Because deep level (stage 4) sleep is so crucial for many body functions, the sleep disorders that frequently occur in fibromyalgia and chronic fatigue patients are thought to be a major contributing factor to the symptoms of this condition. Medicines that help you sleep, control pain and boost your immune system function are commonly prescribed. In addition, non-steroidal, anti-inflammatory drugs (NSAIDs), like ibuprofen, may also be beneficial. Many doctors prescribe trigger point injections with lidocaine, physical therapy, acupuncture, acupressure, relaxation techniques, osteopathic manipulation, chiropractic care, therapeutic massage, or a gentle exercise program. You may want to discuss this menu of treatments with your own physician or health care practitioner.

CHRONIC CONDITIONS

Recipe for self-help:

- Lifestyle modifications may help you conserve your energy and minimize your pain.

- Learn what factors aggravate your symptoms and avoid them, if possible.

- Join a local support group and become informed about your condition.

- Find a health care practitioner who understands this disease and who knows how to treat it to maximize your quality of life.

THYROID PROBLEMS

About half of the 13 million American women who have thyroid disorders don't know it, and many of them feel miserable because of it.

The thyroid gland is a small, butterfly-shaped organ that sits just below the Adam's apple, near the windpipe. It produces hormones that affect nearly every organ, tissue and cell in the body – which is why women suffer so many variable symptoms when the thyroid produces too little hormone (hypothyroidism) or too much (hyperthyroidism). And for reasons not fully understood, women have more thyroid disorders than men. About 1 in 8 women, in fact, will develop a thyroid problem, with the incidence higher among older women, according to the American Medical Women's Association.

The good news is that a fairly simple blood test called a TSH – thyroid stimulating hormone test – can help physicians identify problems before symptoms become severe.

Thyroid cartilage

Thyroid gland

Trachea

Women over 35 are especially encouraged to have regular TSH tests, because thyroid problems are easily treated. Those with too little hormone can be given a synthetic hormone that replaces what the body can't produce. And when the body pumps too much thyroid hormone into the body, doctors can use radioactive iodine to slow it down or remove all or part of the thyroid gland surgically.

What are the symptoms?

HYPOTHYROIDISM (too little thyroid hormone)	HYPERTHYROIDISM (too much thyroid hormone)
Fatigue	Irritability/nervousness
Mood swings	Muscle weakness/tremors
Forgetfulness	Irregular menstrual periods
Weight gain	Weight loss
Dry, coarse skin and hair	Sleep disturbances
Hoarse, froggy voice	Enlarged thyroid (goiter)
Difficulty swallowing	Vision problems or eye irritations
Intolerance to cold	Intolerance to heat

The American Medical Women's Association, which has made thyroid awareness one of its goals, offers this information:

In general, women should be screened with a TSH test if they are over 35, have recently given birth, have high cholesterol or depression, have had thyroid disease in the past or have a history of it, are taking the drugs lithium or amiodarone, have had radiation therapy of the head or neck for cancers or have other autoimmune diseases, such as Addison's disease, Type I diabetes, pernicious anemia, rheumatoid arthritis or lupus.

No matter what kind of chronic condition accompanies you through life, rest assured that you can manage it – whatever it is, from the simplest annoyance to the most severe disease. A lifelong dedication to exercise, a healthful diet, a rich and full social life and healthy interpersonal relationships, combined with a positive attitude and strong communication with your health care team can go a long way to improving your quality of life, no matter what's ahead.

CHAPTER 9

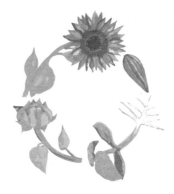

HEART HEALTH

Ask any woman to explain who she is, or to point to the part of her that makes her unique, and watch where her hand moves without fail.

To her brain? Rarely.

To her feet or arms? Hardly ever.

But to her heart? Indeed.

Just as the heart is physically one of the key organs that defines and maintains the human body, it also is the organ which women intuitively feel delineates who they are – as caring individuals, energetic workers, compassionate mothers and loving partners and friends.

Conversely, ask any group of women which disease is most likely to affect their health or lead to their death, and few will intuitively point to the heart. In fact, Dr. Marilyn Gaston, a retired assistant U.S. Surgeon General and preventive health specialist, is continually amazed at how few women know the symptoms of a heart attack or a stroke – or know that heart disease is THE leading killer of women.

Perhaps it's part denial, part rationalization or partly a function of women's busy lives, she speculates. Perhaps women can't fathom how the heart – an organ that intuitively feels so much – can be so troublesome. Indeed, many women are far more worried about breast cancer or other cancers, yet heart disease remains the leading cause of death in women, especially as women pass through mid-life and into the golden years.

The American Heart Association (AHA) is the first to point out the many myths surrounding heart disease – and the critical one is the thinking that heart disease is a "man's disease."

In reality, more women than men die of heart disease. Of all heart-related deaths, 53% occur among women, more than 500,000 a year, or about one death each minute, compared with 46.5% among men, or 440,000 deaths a year. That statistic includes the various types of heart disease, including heart attacks, diseased heart vessels and valves, and stroke.

Consider these statistics about women's hearts:

* 63% of women who die from heart disease had no previous symptoms.
* 42% of women who have heart attacks die within a year, compared to 24% of men.
* During the first six years after a heart attack, the rate of having a second heart attack is 33% for women compared with 21% for men.
* More than half of all women will be affected by heart disease.
* Stroke occurs at a higher rate among African-American and Hispanic women compared with Caucasian women.
* One in four women over age 65 has some form of heart disease.

Here is another sobering fact: after menopause, women's death rates from heart disease are 2-3 times higher than those of women the same age who have not yet reached menopause.

So, as women get older, their risks of heart disease increase exponentially.

Among all population groups – men, women, African-Americans, Caucasians, Hispanics, American Indians and Asian-Pacific Islanders – heart disease is the leading cause of death.

That's why keeping the heart healthy throughout early adulthood and middle age is so important to women – and to their families, friends and spouses.

MAJOR TYPES OF HEART DISEASE

Heart disease isn't one condition or problem. Because the heart is a complicated organ and muscle, the problems that afflict it are also varied and complicated. The purpose of the heart is to pump the blood that bathes every organ of the body. The blood carries oxygen and nutrients to the tissues, and removes waste products from the tissues. If the pumping action of the heart is disrupted, the body's organs begin to fail very quickly. Therefore, life itself is dependent on the efficient operation of the heart.

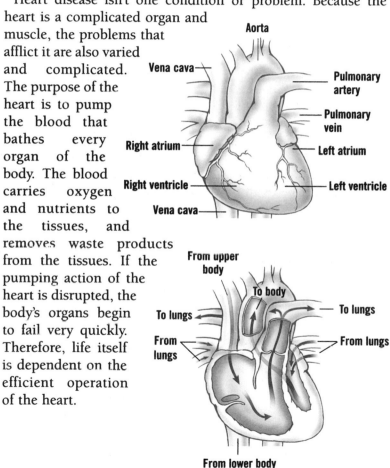

The most common forms of heart disease are:

Blocked arteries or coronary artery disease. This develops when cholesterol and fatty deposits – known as plaque – build up inside the blood vessels, clogging or totally blocking blood flow to the heart muscles or other parts of the body.

Blockages usually develop over time, brought on by a high-fat diet, high blood pressure, cigarette smoking, not exercising and other factors.

Artery wall

Fatty deposit

Clogged Artery

Blood flow

Heart Attack. Also called myocardial infarction, a heart attack occurs when blood flow to the heart is reduced or completely blocked, causing the heart muscles to spasm, degenerate and die.

Angina. This is the medical term for chest pain that results from coronary artery disease, and it's caused by poor circulation and lack of oxygen to the heart.

Congestive Heart Failure. CHF, or heart failure, is a condition in which the heart cannot pump enough blood to the body's other organs. The "failing" heart continues to work, but not as efficiently as it should. The resulting lack of blood flow and oxygen to the body's vital organs causes these organs to begin to fail as well.

Arrhythmia. The heart generates its own electrical signal, or impulse. If the electrical signal becomes erratic in some way, the efficient pumping action of the heart may deteriorate, or stop altogether. This could lead to Sudden Cardiac Death. Abnormal heartbeats can be too fast or too slow. Either way, it is important to see a doctor to determine the cause and for treatment.

Stroke. Women are now urged to think of strokes as "brain attacks," because the process is similar to what happens in a heart attack, though with far different symptoms. In a stroke, blood to the brain is cut off, either because a blood vessel to the brain becomes blocked by plaque or a blood clot (embolus), or because a blood vessel bursts open (aneurysm) and blood gushes into the brain cavity. Deprived of oxygen, the brain shuts down and causes a variety of symptoms throughout the body, including weakness, difficulty speaking or walking. Left untreated, a stroke can lead to coma and death.

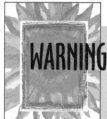

WARNING SIGNS of Stroke

* Weakness in the arms/legs or loss of sensation, usually on one side of the body or face.

* Slurred speech, trouble speaking or understanding what people are saying to you; these symptoms usually get worse over several minutes or hours.

* Double vision or progressive loss of sight, especially in one eye.

* Severe and sudden onset of an excruciating headache.

If you suspect a stroke, call 911 immediately, as many emergency rooms now have stroke teams that can intervene quickly. Quicker treatment generally means a chance for a better long-term outcome and fewer long-term side effects, such as paralysis, slurred speech or one-sided weakness.

High Blood Pressure. Often called the "silent killer" because up to one-third of all people who have high blood pressure don't know it. High blood pressure, or hypertension, is a leading risk factor for a heart attack, stroke or heart failure, according to the AHA. Blood pressure itself is a measure of the pressure inside the blood vessels while the heart pumps and while it is at rest. High blood pressure strains the muscular walls of the blood vessels. High blood pressure is more common and more severe in African-American women. Although the true cause is unknown, high blood pressure can develop because of obesity, smoking and diabetes.

Blood pressure is measured as a reading of two numbers, one on top of the other, such as 120/72. The top number is the **systolic pressure**, or the pressure in the blood vessel when the heart contracts. The bottom number is the **diastolic pressure**, or the pressure inside the blood vessel between contractions. Blood pressure is considered high if the systolic pressure is 140 or higher and the diastolic pressure is 90 or higher.

There are other types of heart disease, including heart valve disease, cardiomyopathy, bacterial infections of the heart muscle or lining, birth defects and more.

IMPORTANT NOTE: Your doctor or cardiologist (heart specialist) is the best person to make any of the above diagnoses. He or she will be able to partner with you to determine which diagnostic tools and treatments will be most effective.

Risk factors for heart disease

Heart disease doesn't start overnight. Some people have a family history of heart disease, putting them more at risk for underlying problems. For many people, heart disease is the result of lifestyle habits and decisions around the issues of diet, activity level, drug and alcohol use and more.

You are at increased risk for heart disease if you:

❀ Smoke cigarettes or use tobacco products.

❀ Are diabetic.

❀ Have high blood pressure.

❀ Are under stress.

❀ Have a family history of heart disease – a sibling or parent who has or had heart problems.

❀ Are not physically active.

❀ Are postmenopausal, as the protective effects of estrogen wear off once estrogen levels fall.

❀ Have high cholesterol, a risk factor that is even more serious in minority populations.

Emerging risk factors?

Just recently, researchers have begun identifying other possible factors for heart disease. While the following are not yet widely tested for, some doctors think that these factors will be included as a normal part of future health exams and checkups.

- One is the "**inflammation factor**," or a swelling reaction that takes place in blood vessels when they become clogged with plaque and fat. Other possible causes for this inflammation could be high blood pressure, smoking and ongoing low-level infections such as chronic gum disease. The body produces a protein – **C-reactive protein (CRP)** – in response to inflammation, and doctors think tests for this protein might be an indicator of future heart disease.

- An amino acid called **homocysteine** might also be a marker for heart disease. Studies are finding that people with high levels of homocysteine have a higher risk of heart disease, stroke and circulatory problems. Elevated levels of this amino acid seem to run in families and individuals whose diets are low in vitamins B6 and B12.

- According to Ginger Graham, former Group Chairman, Office of the President, Guidant Corporation, "Current research now suggests a correlation between calcium build-up in the breast arteries, which may show up in a mammogram, as a risk factor for heart disease." According to researchers, calcifications in three or more breast arteries may be associated with up to a 20% increase in risk for cardiovascular disease.

CHOLESTEROL

Until just recently, doctors focused intensely on the role that cholesterol played in heart disease, and many medicines to lower cholesterol have been developed. With research identifying new risk factors, however, cholesterol is becoming less and less the primary focus of heart disease and is now being viewed as just one more important factor among many in the development of heart disease.

Cholesterol by itself is a waxy, fat-like substance that the body makes naturally to help cells grow and function. The body also gets extra amounts of cholesterol from the foods you eat – mostly animal meats. Too much cholesterol creates blobs of fat that clog arteries and veins, creating the blockages that cause heart disease and stroke. A 25% reduction in total blood cholesterol can cut your risk of heart disease in half.

There's actually "good" cholesterol and "bad" cholesterol, depending on what kind of blood proteins, called lipoproteins, that it attaches to in the body. Bad cholesterol is LDL, or low-density lipoprotein, and it delivers excess cholesterol to the artery walls. Good cholesterol, or HDL, is high-density lipoprotein, and it actually removes the bad cholesterol from the blood stream. **Remember, "L" = Lousy and "H" = Happy.**

* When you get a cholesterol blood test at your doctor's office or lab, be sure to ask about separate HDL and LDL results.

* Anything above 130 LDL is considered high, and 200 or higher is riskiest.

* For HDL, a reading higher than 40 HDL is considered good, and the higher the better because HDL actually reduces your risk of heart disease.

* A blood test also determines levels of triglycerides, which are other types of fat that are made by the liver or derived from foods you eat. Their role in heart disease isn't as profound as a high LDL level, but there is a correlation between high triglyceride levels and low HDL that produces a higher risk of heart disease. A triglyceride reading of less than 200 is desirable, while 200-239 is considered borderline and higher than 240 is considered high risk.

Reducing your risks

Information and self-education are critical to learning about heart disease and taking the necessary steps to take charge and prevent or manage heart disease. Dr. Gaston suggests:

* Learn your family history. Ask about what killed relatives, or who has suffered from heart disease.

* Review each of the risk factors and decide what you can do to change them.

* Start exercising regularly. A 30-minute walk every few days can help begin reducing your risk of heart disease tomorrow. Once you begin, don't stop.

* Adopt an eating plan that's low in fat and rich in fiber, fruits, vegetables and nutrients.

* Quit smoking. (See Chapter 12)

* Keep diabetes and other underlying chronic diseases under control with proper diet, medical care, exercise and other lifestyle modifications.

* Talk with your doctor about your risks and what you can do to improve your health.

* Manage stress in ways that work for you – support groups, yoga, exercise, relaxation tapes, meditation, etc.

Women's hearts....special precautions

As doctors have learned more about heart disease in women, they're finding that not only are the symptoms different, but the tests used to diagnose it should be approached differently in women, too.

Women, of course, frequently ignore the symptoms of heart disease. More than one woman has ended up in an emergency room with a grocery-shopping list still in her pocket and insistent that it's only a little bit of heartburn, not a full-blown

MEN'S SYMPTOMS	WOMEN'S SYMPTOMS
Pressure/fullness/crushing feeling in the chest area	A feeling of breathlessness, often without chest pain of any kind
Difficulty breathing, lightheadedness, fainting	Flu-like symptoms – clammy feeling, nausea, cold sweats
Pain that shoots down one arm or in the jaw	Unexplained fatigue, weakness or dizziness
Nausea	Feelings of anxiety
Sweating	Pain in the upper back, shoulders, neck or jaw; pain can be sudden or it can come and go

heart attack. That's why it's important to KNOW the symptoms that women typically experience. It could be a matter of life and death!

"Don't overlook any of these symptoms," Dr. Gaston emphasizes. "I don't care what you're doing or how busy you are or who you're taking care of. Women need to know about these differences in heart attack symptoms, because they can be life-saving."

If you have a heart attack: Do's and Don'ts

DO NOT assume it's heartburn or stress and that it will go away if you lie down and rest.

DO NOT take a nap and wait for symptoms to subside.

DO NOT call your doctor and wait for hours for a return call. Each minute lost means more heart muscle damaged from lack of blood and oxygen.

DO call 911, alert your family doctor and immediately go to the hospital emergency room.

DO insist that the tests performed are the best ones for women. A simple EKG or treadmill test may not be enough to adequately diagnose your problem. An echocardiogram, angiogram or some kind of nuclear imaging test might be better suited for women's heart disease.

BE PROACTIVE

Reducing heart disease risk means reducing the amount of fat in your diet, and while experts seem to keep changing their minds about what's better – all natural butter or hydrogenated oils in margarine, for example – most experts recommend lowering all types of fats and choosing those that have the kinds of oils most common in the body and are healthiest for the heart.

- **When cooking or frying your food**, choose liquid oils such as olive oil or vegetable oils. Use non-stick cookware or rely on non-stick cooking sprays when you do cook with oil.

- **Trim fat off pieces of meat**, especially chicken and beef. Eat more fatty fish that contain Omega-3 fatty acids: tuna, salmon, mackerel and haddock are good choices.

- **Limit processed foods,** which typically have more fat – snacks, baked goods, anything with palm or coconut oil, salad dressings.
- **Choose low-fat dairy products,** such as cheeses, yogurts, milk and ice cream. Many producers are now making soy milk and ice cream alternatives that are nutritious and tasty.
- **If you have high blood pressure,** take prescribed medicines or treatments to keep it under control.
- **If you have diabetes,** follow a healthy diet and take recommended medicines and treatments to keep blood sugar levels stable.
- **Stress?** Get a grip on stress in your life by exercising or pursuing mind-body strategies that help you relax and keep things in perspective.

IF YOU HAVE experienced a heart attack or underlying disease

- Ask your doctor about taking aspirin daily to prevent future heart attacks or prevent clotting.
- Talk to your doctor about an eating plan and exercise plan that may help you prevent another heart attack.
- Talk to your doctor about new medicines or treatments that can reduce your chance of having another heart attack (or stroke).
- If your problem is an irregular heart beat, talk to your doctor about referring you to a cardiac specialist. This doctor may suggest several options. These may include specific testing, lifestyle modifications or an implantable defibrillator that may regulate the heart's electrical current and keep it stable.

Take care of your heart. Remember, the care you want to give others depends on the care you give to your self.

CHAPTER 10

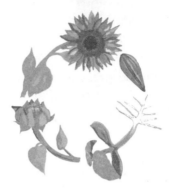

TRUST YOUR GUT

Have you ever had butterflies in your stomach?...Felt a churning sensation in your midsection? Remember that flutter you felt the first time you fell in love?...Sensed your stomach tying itself in knots over something particularly stressful or difficult? Have you ever had the sudden urge to run to the bathroom just before speaking in public or before an important meeting?

The stomach may be the way to a man's heart, but it says a great deal about women, too. In fact, some experts describe the woman's stomach as her "second brain," because it often sends signals – whether we recognize them or not – about intuition, stress, internal problems or health conditions that require our attention.

Indeed, the "gut" can be a barometer of overall emotional and physical health. Women frequently talk about the importance of listening to "female intuition" or "trusting your gut," and the saying has both literal and figurative meanings. Research now shows that there are more neurotransmitters in the 20 feet or so of your "gut" than there are in your brain. So, when you have "butterflies in your stomach," or you just have that "feeling in your gut," it really is a legitimate mind-body connection. **Psychologically**, intuition can be a great thing. **Physiologically**, it can create problems in your gut like heartburn, indigestion and IBS (irritable bowel syndrome).

For some women, chronically upset stomachs may be the body's way of telling us that there are things in life that we just can't "stomach" anymore – unhappy relationships or underlying issues that may need to be explored. Irritable bowel syndrome may be your body's way of telling you that you're holding too much inside, or lacking a sense of control over your world. If women think of the body as a message system, we know what it's trying to tell us only if we take the time to stop, listen and think about the connection between physical symptoms and emotional health.

So let's look at the body's digestive system. Because it's major job is to digest the food you eat, the stomach is a churning cauldron of acids and chemicals that break food down into a mushy form so that it can pass into the intestines, where key nutrients are absorbed into the bloodstream. Food that's chewed in the mouth enters into the esophagus, a muscular tube about nine or so inches long. At the top of the esophagus is a small valve that relaxes to let food enter the esophagus and to keep it from going where it's not supposed to go, or "down the wrong pipe"...also known as down the trachea to the lungs.

At the bottom of the esophagus is a stronger valve that relaxes to let food into the stomach. When the lower valve fails to work properly, food backs up into the esophagus causing a variety of symptoms that cause heartburn.

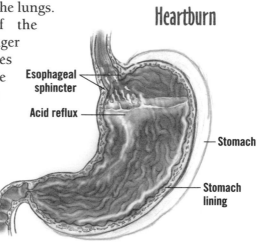

Heartburn

Esophageal sphincter

Acid reflux

Stomach

Stomach lining

The Gut Anatomy

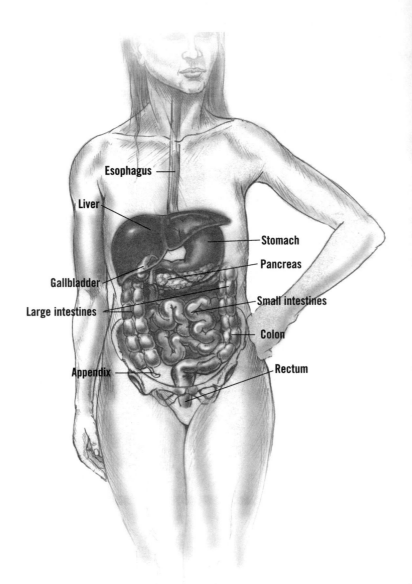

119

HEARTBURN

One of the most common ailments is heartburn, named because it feels as if the heart just inside or below the rib cage is on fire. In reality, this condition has nothing to do with your heart. But heartburn is a common occurrence, affecting an estimated 44% of the population. And even though it's common, only about 25% of the people who suffer from heartburn seek medical help for their problems.

Heartburn experts urge women similarly to "trust their gut" when they begin experiencing stomach problems or symptoms of heartburn. Typically, it's the body's way of sending a message that something is out of kilter and needs to be addressed.

What happens is that the stomach acids that are hard at work digesting food can back up from the stomach into the esophagus, and because acid is irritating, it causes a burning sensation in the chest and above the rib cage. Heartburn causes a variety of symptoms:

* A "burning" sensation in the upper chest
* Coughing
* Laryngitis
* Constant throat clearing
* Spasms of the esophagus

Heartburn or Heart Attack?

Some women, in fact, mistake heartburn symptoms for angina or a heart attack, and, even scarier, may mistake a heart attack for heartburn. Symptoms can be similar, and if there is the slightest question, **please, please seek medical attention immediately!**

Heartburn and upset stomachs take an emotional toll as well. You may not be able to eat the foods you want or enjoy the activities that bring pleasure – gardening or biking or exercise, for example. You may wake up in the middle of the night and experience restlessness and fatigue the rest of the day. You may feel trapped inside your house, always wondering when the next bout of heartburn will strike, or when you go out socially, you may worry constantly or refrain from enjoying food.

Some health conditions and medical situations can cause heartburn or worsen its effects. They include:

Pregnancy: As the fetus grows, so does the uterus, pushing on organs. Its increasing size can begin to squish organs and squeeze contents of the stomach back into the esophagus. Usually, pregnant women are advised to eat smaller, more frequent meals during the day and to avoid large meals.

Gastroesophageal Reflux Disease (GERD): GERD is a chronic form of heartburn, especially if it occurs several times a week. The irritating acids that creep back into the esophagus can cause tissue in the esophagus to redden, swell and become permanently damaged. Left untreated, it can cause so much damage to the esophagus that the cellular damage may lead to cancer.

Hiatal hernia: This is a common cause of GERD, that occurs when the muscular valve that controls the flow of contents from the esophagus to the stomach doesn't close fully, allowing part of the stomach to poke back up into the esophagus. According to the *Johns Hopkins Family Medical Health Book*, about 40% of the population has a hiatal hernia with no symptoms, but if problems are severe, doctors may have to perform surgery to repair it.

Diabetes: This disorder affects the body's ability to produce or use insulin, and can cause nausea and vomiting that mimic heartburn symptoms. (See Chapter 8)

Certain medicines: These include aspirin, pain-relievers, some antibiotics, some osteoporosis medicines, vitamins and iron tablets, and may irritate the digestive tract and create heartburn-like symptoms. Read labels and instructions on whether medicine should or should not be taken with food.

Treating heartburn

Often, taking care of heartburn doesn't have to involve complicated medical treatments. The National Heartburn Alliance and other health professionals recommend some simple lifestyle changes that can drastically improve digestive health and reduce symptoms.

* **First, quit smoking.** Nicotine and the other damaging components in tobacco can upset your metabolism and throw the stomach chemicals out of balance. Even after quitting, it may take several weeks or months for digestion to return to normal.

* **Lose weight.** Like many other common health problems, carrying too much weight on the body can force it to work harder to perform simple functions, and digestion is one of them. Just the mere act of lying down as an overweight person can put tremendous pressure on the stomach and digestive organs. Losing weight takes a load off, literally and figuratively.

* **Wear loose-fitting clothes.** You might want to squeeze into something a size smaller, but tight waistbands, belts and other constrictive clothes may make the heartburn symptoms worse. Look for pantyhose that are just your size.

* **Don't rush meals.** Enjoy each bite. Slow down. Relax while you eat. If you take time to chew food slowly and savor each morsel, you'll relax other organs internally and make it easier for digestion to take place naturally, without all the churning and burning.

* **Avoid overeating.** Eating too much can trigger heartburn, as there simply isn't room in the digestive system for all that food, and it has nowhere to go but backwards. Remember, your stomach can be full 20-30 minutes before your brain recognizes the "full" feeling that normally tells you it's time to put down the fork.

* **Don't eat right before bedtime.** Lying down can cause stomach acids to back up, which is why some people experience heartburn at night.

* **"Fight acid creep while you sleep."** That's the slogan used by The National Heartburn Alliance in its recommendation to raise the head of your bed 4-6

inches by placing blocks or bricks underneath the bed's legs, or try something as simple as elevating your head and shoulders 4-6 inches by using an extra pillow. Doing so may prevent acid from creeping up into the esophagus and uses the well-known effects of gravity to keep it in the stomach, where it belongs.

⊛ **Know your medications.** Some medicines can cause digestion problems. Be sure to read labels and talk over all your medicines – prescription and over-the-counter – with your doctor or pharmacist.

Avoid Trigger Foods

Some foods naturally contain more acid than others or, once eaten, trigger its production in the stomach. Do you know which ones are troublesome for you? Keeping a food diary will help you pay attention to foods that are most likely to set off your heartburn symptoms. Try to avoid them in the future.

Common foods linked to heartburn may include:
  ⊛ Fatty or spicy foods
  ⊛ Carbonated beverages
  ⊛ Peppermint or spearmint
  ⊛ Citrus fruits
  ⊛ Tomatoes
  ⊛ Whole milk
  ⊛ Coffee
  ⊛ Onions

Source: *Johns Hopkins Family Health Book*

*Chocolate – a word about chocolate…unfortunately, in some people, chocolate may be a trigger. But, since many of us as women consider chocolate "an essential food group," Robin Miller, M.D., suggests eating a small **piece** of chocolate, instead of a small **box**!*

If lifestyle changes aren't enough to keep heartburn at bay, several types of medicines are available. They work on the same principles: reducing the amount of acid that the stomach and esophagus are exposed to in order to reduce the likelihood of setting off the burning sensations and other symptoms.

The most common medicines are:

Over-the-counter antacids, such as Tums, Maalox, Rolaids and Mylanta, neutralize the acid in the stomach and are good for relieving symptoms quickly. The liquid forms work fast, but some people may consider tablets more convenient. The drawback is that the effect of these antacids may not last long, so repeating doses may be required for relief.

Over-the-counter and prescription H2 blockers, such as Pepcid AC and Zantac, work by blocking histamine receptors (that's what H2 stands for). These receptors stimulate the production of the stomach acids, and by blocking them, the stomach makes less acid, reducing the likelihood of heartburn.

Proton Pump Inhibitors (PPI), such as the newer prescription drugs Prilosec, Prevacid and Nexium, are powerful substances that block or suppress acid production in the cells that "pump" acid into the stomach. Some studies also find that they may decrease heartburn-related symptoms, including shortness of breath, hoarseness, chronic cough and laryngitis. Remember, these are medications in pill form, and not an actual pump. Once the drugs are at work, they may relieve or prevent symptoms for up to 24 hours.

Other Prescription Drugs: Doctors also have access to so-called prokinetic medicines that may heal the painful swelling in the esophagus, and which are typically prescribed for long-term use. Other drugs may speed up digestion, keeping food in the stomach for shorter periods of time so that reflux has less of a chance to occur, while still others may protect the mucous lining of the esophagus to keep it healthy and functioning.

As with all drug treatments, talk with your doctor or pharmacist about risks, benefits and possible side effects.

In severe cases of GERD or hiatal hernia, doctors might have to perform surgery to repair the valves that control the flow of contents and acid between the stomach and esophagus.

Herbal or supplemental remedies

Dr. Andrew Weil, well-known author and integrative medicine specialist at the University of Arizona, recommends several supplements for indigestion and heartburn-like symptoms. They include:

DGL, which stands for deglycyrrhizinated licorice, can soothe indigestion by increasing the mucous lining of the esophagus. Chewable tablets may provide quick relief, and maybe this is why our grandmothers always had little licorice pills on the nightstand.

Slippery elm, an herbal remedy, may also soothe and protect the mucous tissue of the esophagus.

Chamomile, as a tea or an extract, may calm the stomach.

Remember to consider any herbal supplements as "medications." If your doctor asks, "what medications are you taking?" be sure to include over-the-counter and herbal supplements in your answer. Also ask your doctor or pharmacist if there is a reason not to mix herbs and/or over-the-counter medications with your prescription drugs.

IRRITABLE BOWEL SYNDROME

If you've ever had Irritable Bowel Syndrome, it can be as nasty as it sounds. It usually means that women experience abdominal pain or discomfort and accompanying changes in bowel patterns.

For some, loose stools and frequent bowel movements may become the norm. For others, diarrhea develops and never seems to go away, while some women develop constipation.

Usually, doctors discuss symptoms and try to rule out other problems, such as gallbladder disease or cancers. Once a diagnosis is made, the doctor and patient develop a plan that works. The good news is that lifestyle and dietary changes can typically bring about tremendous relief.

TRUST YOUR GUT

Some simple things can keep IBS at bay:

Keep a diary of what factors bring on IBS symptoms. Certain foods? Certain emotional events or stresses? Try to determine what lifestyle changes **you** can make to regain a sense of control and order in your life.

Try relaxation techniques or hypnosis to calm the entire body and restore normal bowel movements and functions. Stress can be a large factor in IBS, and biofeedback is used to control stress for many common health problems. Sometimes biofeedfback can also be used to help calm and pay attention to the body's rhythms and patterns.

Change what you eat. Keep track of certain foods that tend to set off your IBS. Common foods that are linked to IBS vary widely, but might include citrus fruits or juices, potatoes, onions, garlic, cabbage, green beans, broccoli, milk products, breads or grains, cheeses, meats, eggs and nuts. Other foods or substances that can upset digestion and metabolism include alcohol, nicotine, coffee, tea and chocolate.

For severe symptoms, doctors may recommend several drugs developed specifically for IBS, and sometimes women are also urged to take low-dose antidepressants for pain. Professionals at the International Foundation for Functional Gastrointestinal Disorders point out that medicines, however, should be used in conjunction with other lifestyle changes and approaches, not in place of them.

CONSTIPATION

It's not something that women like to talk about, but constipation can be more than just uncomfortable and upsetting. If it continues long-term, it also can be a risk factor for more serious problems, including hemorrhoids and various intestinal diseases. Simply defined, constipation means difficulty having a bowel movement, usually because stools become too hard or have difficulty passing out of the body.

Usually, some simple remedies can solve most problems with constipation.

⊛ Drink plenty of fluids, at least 8 glasses of water a day.

- Eat high-fiber foods, at least 40 grams a day, recommends Dr. Andrew Weil. Good sources of fiber include high-fiber cereals, fresh vegetables, fruits and legumes, such as beans and peas.

- Fiber supplements, such as psyllium, can help keep bowels moving regularly, but make sure to drink plenty of fluids with these products.

- Exercise also tones the intestines and tissues that keep digested food moving through the body. Try taking a walk after meals or on a regular basis. Even something as simple as a walk can get muscles moving in a more normal pattern.

- If you're stressed, try some sort of daily relaxation technique, such as meditation, deep breathing, yoga or a relaxation tape. Being "uptight" is more than just a frame of mind. Tightened, stressed muscles can also lead to problems such as constipation.

- Pay attention to your body's normal rhythms and cycles and try to accommodate them as much as possible. Fighting the urge to "go" can just make the problem worse, because the longer that stools stay in the bowel, the more liquid they lose, making them harder and more difficult to pass out of the body.

Remember, your body sends messages of all kinds, and it's always important to pay attention! Trust your intuition, and trust your gut!

CHAPTER 11

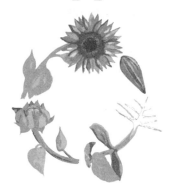

BONE HEALTH

Would you believe, this year in the United States, more women will suffer a hip fracture than will be diagnosed with breast, ovarian and uterine cancer combined? Think a hip fracture is no big deal? Think again. A hip fracture almost always requires hospitalization and major surgery. It can impair a person's ability to walk unassisted and may cause permanent disability or even death!

For the bone-thinning disease known as osteoporosis, a seemingly simple act such as a trip or a fall can be a significant, life-altering trigger that makes women aware just how fragile their bones are.

"People may not know that they have osteoporosis until their bones become so weak that a sudden strain, bump or fall causes a fracture or a vertebra to collapse," according to the National Osteoporosis Foundation (NOF).

Indeed, of the 10 million Americans who have osteoporosis at any one time, 8 million of them are women. It's a disease whose incidence increases as women age, and all ethnic backgrounds are at risk. While osteoporosis is often thought of as an older person's disease, it can strike at any age.

The NOF notes that one in two women over age 50 will experience an osteoporosis-related fracture at some time in their life. Each year, in fact, Americans experience 300,000 hip fractures and more than twice as many spinal fractures.

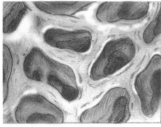

Healthy bone

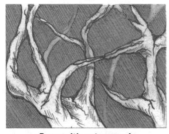

Bone with osteoporois

"Osteoporosis is primarily a woman's disease, because it is heavily influenced by the hormones that fluctuate in a woman's body throughout life," explains Lana Holstein, M.D. Estrogen protects the bones of younger and middle-aged women, bones that must be built with adequate minerals, calcium, Vitamin D and nutrients throughout life to remain healthy into the golden years. Once estrogen drops during the menopausal years, the body begins to draw calcium and minerals from the bone, making them porous rather than solid and firm. As bones weaken, women are at greater risk of fractures of the spine, wrist, hip and ankle.

"Women are at great risk from osteoporosis," notes Holstein, "because they watch their calories and don't necessarily make sure they have enough calcium and vitamins in their diet and don't necessarily do those weight-bearing exercises."

SWH National Honorary Chair, actress & co-host of Lifetime's Speaking of Women's Health, Florence Henderson, says "Many women who have been conscientious about taking calcium supplements and having adequate calcium in their diets as well as maintaining a regular weight-bearing exercise program, such as walking and lifting weights, are shocked to find that they have osteoporosis. The only way to know for sure if you have osteoporosis is to see your doctor and have a DEXA screening. This was exactly my experience. After my DEXA screening, my doctor put me on a medicine and recent screenings show improvement."

BONE HEALTH

ARE YOU AT RISK?

The more you answer "yes" to the following factors, the greater your risk for osteoporosis:

* You have a family history of osteoporosis (relatives with stooped posture or broken bones, frequent fractures).

* You eat a diet low in calcium and Vitamin D.

* You have low bone mass, as indicated by bone-density tests.

* You don't do weight-bearing exercises regularly – walking, hiking, stair climbing, jogging, skiing, aerobic dancing, training with hand weights or larger weights.

* You smoke cigarettes.

* You are of Caucasian or Asian heritage.

* You have a small or thin body structure.

* You are past menopause (naturally or because of surgery); in the 5-7 years after menopause, women can lose up to 20% of their bone mass.

* You consume alcohol excessively.

* You have taken oral steroids, thyroid medicine or anti-convulsant drugs for a long time.

* You have the eating disorder known as anorexia nervosa.

* You take more than 700 mg a day of Vitamin A, now thought to increase a woman's risk of bone fractures.

How do you know if have osteoporosis?

A disease like osteoporosis can exist without symptoms, so women may have weak or thinning bones and not know it. A bone densitometry or DEXA is a state-of-the art radiology test that can determine the bone mass or density of bone minerals. This simple, painless test usually takes 15 minutes or less and delivers only a small amount of radiation to the body. A woman usually lies on an X-ray machine while an arm moves slowly over her pelvis and hips. Once the test is finished, the results are reviewed by a radiologist and can be a useful tool for your doctor in diagnosing and treating osteoporosis, especially in the early stages before fractures or broken bones occur. The test results are measured as "T Scores."

What the T Score Means

* A T Score of –1.0 or higher means you have normal bones and a low risk of osteoporosis. Keep up the good work!

* A T Score of –1.0 to –2.5 means you have a medium risk of osteoporosis with a low bone mass. It's time to take action!

* A T Score of –2.5 or lower means you have a high risk of osteoporosis and bones that are weak and prone to breaking or fracture. Talk to your health care professional now!

Treating Osteoporosis

There is no cure for osteoporosis, but women can begin in their early adult and middle years to build strong bones that will last into the golden years. Even when osteoporosis risks are high, women can institute lifestyle, dietary and medical measures to slow down bone loss or reduce (as much as possible) the risks of a bone break or fracture. The National Osteoporosis Foundation urges these steps for treating the disease:

* Do your utmost to build strong bones before the age of 30 through regular exercise, adequate calcium and Vitamin D intake, and calcium supplements if necessary. Many foods today now have calcium added to them – juices, cereals, breakfast bars and the like. Take advantage of ready-made, easy-to-eat foods that have all the vitamins and nutrients you need!

* Follow a diet rich in calcium and Vitamin D.

* Adopt an exercise program that includes weight-bearing exercises several times a week. This can be as simple as walking…you are bearing your own body weight.

* Do not smoke. Use alcohol in moderate amounts only.

* Undergo bone density testing and take necessary medications when appropriate.

BONE HEALTH

Calcium and Vitamin D are friends

Calcium is necessary to build and maintain strong bones and muscles, but the body can't absorb calcium without the help of Vitamin D. And if you've ever noticed, you can't buy Vitamin D pills at the drug store. Vitamin D's two primary sources are direct exposure to the sunlight and from fortified dairy products, egg yolks, saltwater fish and liver. Many milk products today have Vitamin D added to them. Be sure to choose a calcium supplement that contains Vitamin D and magnesium to ensure adequate absorption.

How much calcium? Women need adequate levels of calcium, a finding that is especially true for African-American women. The NIH estimates that many African-American women get less than half the amount of calcium recommended. For women who cannot tolerate dairy products, calcium supplements and calcium chew tabs are a possible alternative.

The National Academy of Sciences recommends these levels of calcium for women. As your body can only absorb 600 mg of calcium at a time, be sure to take your supplements in divided doses.

AGE	CALCIUM PER DAY	VITAMIN D PER DAY
9-18	1300 mg	
19-50 (premenopausal)	1000 mg	400-800 IU
51 and older	1200 mg	every day

Medical treatment

The U.S Food and Drug Administration has approved several medicines for preventing or treating osteoporosis. They fall into several categories.

Bisphosphonates make up one group, and they include drugs such as alendronate and risedronate. Taken in pill form, both can irritate the esophagus, so women are urged not to lie down for at least 30 minutes after taking the drugs.

Other types include polypeptides, prescription estrogen or hormone replacement therapy and selective estrogen receptor modulators. Not all drugs are equal or offer the same benefits.

Ask your doctor which will work best for you and help reduce your risk of bone fracture, particularly hip and spine, fastest. As with all prescription drugs, talk with your doctor about benefits, risks and possible side effects.

THE FRACTURE EQUATION

For many women, the real devastation of osteoporosis occurs when they slip, fall or trip and fracture a bone – usually the hip or an arm or leg bone. The problems are amplified among older women, who may take longer to recover or never fully walk again after a broken hip.

Hip Joint

Femoral neck

Pelvis

Femur

"During the year after a woman has a hip fracture, nearly 20% will die," notes Lana Holstein, M.D., "because a fracture like that is a trauma that sets up a reaction throughout the body, and may cause pneumonia, heart attacks, strokes and other conditions that are associated with treatment and bedrest because of the fracture."

That's why preventing osteoporosis – and the resulting fractures – is a key focus of the health care approach today.

The National Institutes of Health identifies "The Fracture Triangle" as a three-factor approach to thinking about broken bones.

Fall

THE FRACTURE TRIANGLE

Force   Fragility

If any of these three factors is lessened or improved, the chances of breaking a bone are greatly reduced. Let's take a look at what's involved in the triangle.

The Fall. The act of falling can be caused by tripping, losing traction, slipping or losing one's footing over something unseen. Women can reduce the risks of falling by doing muscle-strengthening exercises, making sure contact lens and eyeglass prescriptions are updated, and practicing balancing and reaction exercises. Yoga is also very good for retaining balance, posture, stability and strength. Practice falling by slumping onto a bed and rolling into a ball, rather than stiffening and using arms/legs to break your fall.

The Force. How hard a person lands, and in what direction, can determine whether bones are broken or fractured. The greater the distance to the floor, the greater the risk of breaking a hip. Falling sideways or straight down is more risky than falling backwards, according to the NIH. Learning how to react to a fall can help reduce its severity. Grabbing for something with your hand, for example, might fracture a wrist but will spare a more devastating hip fracture. Hip pads, sewn into special undergarments, also can reduce the risk of a hip fracture.

Fragility. Bones that were once strong can become so weak and fragile that they break easily from even the slightest movement or bump. Getting enough calcium and Vitamin D, exercising several times a week, getting bone-density tests and talking to your doctor about medicines that strengthen the bones can help reduce fragility and the risk of fractures.

Spine

Hip

Wrist

Bone health guidelines

Look at what the National Osteoporosis Foundation has to say about understanding the health of your bones. It is important to understand that bone is not a hard and lifeless structure. It is, in fact, a complex, living tissue. Our bones provide structural support for muscles, protect vital organs, and store the calcium essential for bone density and strength.

Because bones are constantly changing, they can heal and may be affected by diet and exercise. Until the age of about 30, you build and store bone efficiently. Then, as part of the natural aging process, your bones begin to break down faster than new bone can be formed. In women, bone loss accelerates after menopause, when your ovaries stop producing estrogen. Think of your bones as a savings account. There is only as much bone mass in your account as you deposit. The critical years for building bone mass are from prior to adolescence to about age 30. Some experts believe that young women can increase their bone mass by as much as 20 percent – a critical factor in protecting against osteoporosis.

Assessing your bone health

To determine if you have osteoporosis or may be at risk for the disease, your doctor will ask you a variety of questions about your lifestyle and medical history. Your doctor will want to know if anyone in your family has suffered from osteoporosis or if they have fractured bones. Based on a comprehensive medical assessment, your doctor may recommend that you have your bone mass measured.

A bone mass measurement is the only way to tell if you have osteoporosis. Specialized tests called bone density tests can measure bone density in various sites of the body. A bone density test can:

* Detect osteoporosis before a fracture occurs.

* Predict your chances of fracturing in the future.

* Determine your rate of bone loss and/or monitor the effects of treatment if the test is conducted at intervals of a year of more.

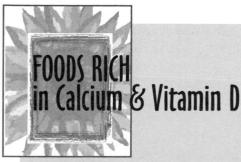

FOODS RICH in Calcium & Vitamin D

Calcium

- Dairy foods such as milk, cheese, yogurt and ice cream
- Calcium-added cereals, breakfast bars, breads and orange juice
- Mozzarella, ricotta, cheddar, Swiss, cottage and parmesan cheeses
- Canned salmon with bones and sardines
- Navy beans
- Nuts
- Tofu
- Turnips, kale, broccoli, leafy green vegetables
- Blackstrap molasses

Vitamin D

Food sources of Vitamin D include fatty fish (salmon, mackerel) and fish oils. Milk and other foods are often fortified with Vitamin D, but products made from milk such as cheese, yogurt, etc. are not necessarily fortified and may not contain Vitamin D. Check the label. Exposure to sunlight is also a source of Vitamin D, and an important component of your body's ability to absorb calcium.

CHAPTER 12

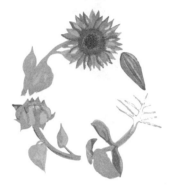

QUIT SMOKING NOW
For A Better Life To Come!

Every single day, millions of American women follow a predictable routine. First, they reach into a purse, briefcase or drawer for a pack of cigarettes. Pull one out. Tap it lightly on a flat surface. Reach for a lighter, flick the dial and light up a cigarette – knowing full well that it contains some of the most addictive and dangerous substances to their health.

And just as predictably, millions of American women **successfully quit smoking, too.**

The U.S. Surgeon General's report on smoking in 1964 was the first wake-up call to stop smoking cigarettes. In fact, it was the first public announcement that smoking was potentially deadly.

Decades later, the ammunition against smoking has only increased – but the hard job of quitting smoking hasn't changed since 1964. It's just as difficult today as it was then. But, we have plenty of reasons to try.

Smoking-related diseases kill 440,000 Americans a year from a variety of diseases now linked to smoking. They include lung

QUIT SMOKING NOW For A Better Life To Come!

cancer, heart disease, stroke, chronic lung disease and emphysema, chronic asthma, mouth and throat cancer, bladder and kidney cancer, pancreatic cancer, osteoporosis and more. If that's not enough reason, consider that smoking also affects your beauty and skin health. Drawing on the cigarette with your lips causes unnatural wrinkles to develop around your mouth.

For women, the consequences are far-reaching.

❧ Lung cancer kills more women than any other cancer each year, and the vast majority of all lung cancer deaths are smoking-related. In fact, women over 35 who smoke are 12 times more likely to die prematurely from lung cancer than women who don't smoke. According to the Harvard Nurses' Health Study, just 1-4 cigarettes a day can double a woman's risk of heart attack. Smoking is also related to cervical cancer in women.

❧ Smoking during pregnancy, while trying to become pregnant or while raising infants and young children also takes a toll. Pregnant women who smoke have a higher rate of complications during pregnancy, are more likely to deliver babies who are underweight and are more prone to sickness and early death. Smoking during pregnancy may increase the risk of experiencing a miscarriage or a stillbirth.

❧ Smokers who use oral contraceptives are at increased risk of stroke, heart disease and potentially fatal blood clots.

❧ Children exposed to second-hand smoke are at higher risk for asthma and chronic bronchitis, frequent colds, ear infections and sudden infant death syndrome. According to research, even family pets face a higher risk of cancers from inhaling second-hand smoke.

Why quit smoking?

Over the years, the evidence against smoking has mounted, but today, there are more and more reasons to quit…and more effective methods of actually kicking the smoking habit.

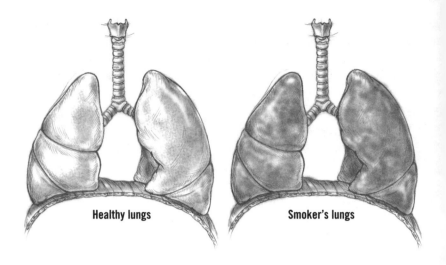

Healthy lungs   Smoker's lungs

Reasons to quit are plenty, especially if you're a Can-Do Woman who wants to make decisions that are healthy, life-prolonging, vital and reaffirming.

SMOKING IS AN ADDICTION

Smoking addiction has two components. First, there's a physical and psychological dependence on nicotine. The body craves nicotine and undergoes withdrawal symptoms when it doesn't get it regularly – a true sign of addiction. Smoking also involves a lifestyle component, or a habit. Smoking becomes a ritual associated with everyday tasks such as talking on the phone or taking a 15-minute smoke break.

Habits are formed by repetition. A pack-a-day smoker repeats the hand-to-mouth ritual of lighting and puffing on a cigarette about 200 times a day. That's 73,000 times a year. In addition, some smokers seem to associate the feel, smell and sight of a cigarette – as well as the rituals of getting, handling, lighting, and smoking the cigarette – with the pleasurable effects of smoking. When these smokers try to quit, this association can make the symptoms of withdrawal or craving worse.

A new report on smoking cessation and gender, published in February 2003, suggests that women smokers may have a higher behavioral dependence on cigarettes and a lower nicotine dependence than men. Women may be more inclined to the habit of repetitive actions of smoking than are men. While both men and women are addicted to the nicotine in cigarettes, successful cessation may require behavioral modification in the form of hand-to-mouth habit replacement.

"Our study showed that women appear to have higher behavioral and lower nicotine dependence than men," said study lead author Abraham Bohadana, M.D., Research Director, French National Institute of Health. "A nicotine inhaler may be a good tool for women as it not only provides nicotine craving relief but also seems to satisfy the 'hand to mouth' habit smokers are used to."

Knowing that counsel and support may further increase a smoker's chances of quitting, those who want to quit should also utilize behavior and support programs, such as the American Cancer Society's Break Away from the Pack. Another place to look for information is www.speakingofwomenshealth.com.

Physically, the reasons to quit are numerous. Quitting means confronting and dealing with the dependence on nicotine and finding other habits or making lifestyle changes to accommodate something to take its place.

Nicotine does more than give you a temporary "buzz" or feeling of euphoria. In fact, the components in cigarettes – and there are thousands of them, many of them poisonous – affect nearly every organ and system in your body. And none of the effects are good ones. Some experts believe that the most harmful effects of smoking are not caused by nicotine itself, but by the 4,000 other chemicals in tobacco smoke, including more than 40 known cancer-causing agents. Let's take a look.

Brain

When you smoke: Within 7 seconds of inhaling smoke, feel-good chemicals called endorphins are released, stimulating pleasurable feelings and masking pain. Cells that attract nicotine molecules increase, creating cravings and addictive sensations.

When you stop: You'll feel temporarily grouchy and blue, because your body has to learn to manufacture its own endorphins naturally, again. Try exercise, laughter, relaxation, physical contact and walking to recharge your body!

Temperament

When you smoke: Your body's ability to absorb caffeine is blocked.

When you quit: You'll have to cut back on caffeine because the amount you consumed while smoking will deliver a bigger-than-normal jolt.

Lungs

When you smoke: Lung cells turn red, swell, harden and die as smoke robs them of needed oxygen. Eventually, breathing becomes difficult and lung cells can turn cancerous.

When you quit: Swollen, red lung cells begin to improve and heal. Lung function can return to normal in about three months.

Heart

When you smoke: Smoke and its by-products rob the heart of oxygen, triggering the production of plaque and clogged arteries. Blood pressure increases as the heart works harder to oxygenate and circulate blood to the rest of the body. Hands and feet turn cold, as blood flow is restricted.

When you quit: The heart beats easier with enough oxygen to do its job, blood pressure declines and arteries clear out naturally. Sensations of warmth return to the hands and feet. Heart health may return to normal in about two years.

QUIT SMOKING NOW For A Better Life To Come!

Stomach
When you smoke: Cigarettes trigger the production of stomach acid, which can lead to heartburn and digestive problems. It also raises metabolism, so you digest food more quickly.

When you stop: Digestive system and metabolism may be temporarily off balance when you quit, causing temporary "blah" feelings, upset stomach and slight weight gain. Drink plenty of fluids, exercise, and eat lots of fiber. The benefits will "outweigh" this issue.

Skin
When you smoke: Carbon monoxide takes the place of oxygen in the blood, slowing circulation to skin cells and causing wrinkles and crow's feet. Without needed oxygen and hemoglobin, skin also becomes paler and ashen.

When you quit: Oxygenated blood flows to skin again, slowing the development of wrinkles and premature aging and restoring a healthier skin tone and color.

Sexuality
When you smoke: Reduced blood flow to critical organs can cause impotence in men and slowed sexual response in women.

When you quit: Normalized blood flow energizes sexual drive and performance.

Five Common Myths
1.) **Myth: Smoking is just a bad habit.**
   Fact: Tobacco use is an addiction. For some people, it can be as addictive as heroin or cocaine.

2.) **Myth: Quitting is just a matter of willpower.**
   Fact: Because smoking is an addiction, quitting is often very difficult. A number of treatments are available that can help.

3.) **Myth: If you can't quit the first time you try, you will never be able to quit.**
   Fact: Quitting is hard. Usually people make two or three tries, or more, before being able to quit for good.

142

4.) Myth: The best way to quit is "cold turkey."
Fact: The most effective way to quit smoking is by using a combination of counseling and nicotine replacement therapy (such as a nicotine inhaler, patch, gum, or nasal spray) or non-nicotine medicines (such as bupropion SR). Look for nationally-known, pharmacist-recommended products from companies who support education and research about smoking cessation.

5.) Myth: Quitting is expensive.
Fact: Treatments cost from $3 to $10 a day. A pack-a-day smoker spends almost $1,000 per year. How would you prefer to spend your money...for your health or for your addiction?

Get medication and use it correctly

- Medications can help you stop smoking and lessen the urge to smoke.
- The US Food and Drug Administration (FDA) has approved five medications to help you quit smoking.
- Ask your health care provider for advice and carefully read the information on the package.
- All of these medications will more or less double your chances of quitting and quitting for good.
- Everyone who is trying to quit may benefit from using a medication. If you are pregnant or trying to become pregnant, nursing, under age 18, smoking fewer than 10 cigarettes per day, or have a medical condition, talk to your doctor or other health care provider before taking medications.

WHEN YOU QUIT

Shortness of breath, edginess, coughing....all of the physical reactions your body develops from smoking are evidence that your body is working hard to fight the effects of smoke, nicotine and all the other dangerous substances in cigarettes.

QUIT SMOKING NOW For A Better Life To Come!

Here's what the American Cancer Society has to say about how quickly your body begins to recover after quitting:

- **20 minutes after quitting**...blood pressure drops to a level similar to what it was before you lit up the last cigarette. The temperature in your hands and feet returns to normal.

- **8 hours after quitting**...carbon monoxide levels in the blood return to normal.

- **24 hours after quitting**...your chance of a heart attack begins to decrease.

- **2 weeks-3 months after quitting**...blood circulation improves, and lung function increases up to 30%.

- **1-9 months after quitting**...coughing, sinus congestion, fatigue and shortness of breath decrease; the tiny hairs that work in your lungs to catch foreign particles return to normal function, increasing the lungs' ability to handle mucous, clean the lungs and reduce the risk of infection.

- **1 year after quitting**...the risk of heart disease is half that of someone who continues to smoke.

- **5-15 years after quitting**...the risk of having a stroke is reduced to that of a non-smoker.

- **10 years after quitting**...the death rate from lung cancer is about half that of someone who continues to smoke; the risk of cancers of the mouth, throat, esophagus, bladder, kidney and pancreas decrease.

- **15 years after quitting**...the risk of heart disease is similar to that of a non-smoker.

Ways to Quit Smoking

- **Learn new skills and behaviors.** Try to distract yourself from urges to smoke. Talk to someone, go for a walk, or get busy with a new task.
- **When you first try to quit, change your routine.** Take a different route to work. Drink tea instead of coffee. Eat breakfast in a different place.
- **Do something to reduce stress.** Take a hot bath, exercise or read a book.
- **Plan something enjoyable to do every day.**
- **Drink a lot of water and other fluids.**

CHAPTER
13

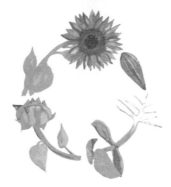

MENTAL HEALTH AND WELLNESS

What makes each individual unique is an awesome blend of mind, body and spirit. Not only is this what makes us unique, it is the key to our mental health and wellness.

Mental and physical health go hand in hand, and medical experts increasingly recognize the critical links between sound mental health and the physical health benefits that accompany it.

Modern society and our culture have placed tremendous importance on physical health, sometimes at the expense of mental health. Even today, some people attach a stigma to people who suffer from very common mental disorders or mental health challenges.

The good news for today's modern woman is that the stigma is rapidly dissolving, thanks to public education programs and open discussions about topics that can range from a celebrity's public bout with depression to legislative debates about insurance coverage for mental health treatment. And more and more treatments are emerging, including prescription drugs, over-the-counter herbal remedies, talk therapies, exercise programs, counseling endeavors and nutritional programs that can either combat symptoms of mental disorders or help lessen them enough that other treatments become more effective.

DEPRESSION

For women, depression is one of the most common mental health problems they face, whether it's depression that sets in during adolescence or after the birth of a baby or later in life, when changes and losses become more difficult to bear. Of course, every one gets "blue" or "down in the dumps" occasionally, but depression is a clinical diagnosis that's made when moods change and stay low for long periods of time.

The important thing to know is that many mental health problems are common and treatable. They're not "all in your head" or easily defeated by "mind over matter" or some deep-down source of untapped will power. Depression itself is a legitimate, treatable disease, one with very real symptoms and solutions.

Indeed, some people who battle depression say it feels as if they're fogged in by a thick cloud, or stuck swimming upstream, struggling against an unseen but heavy presence.

A Personal Story...

This is how one woman in her 60s described how her lifelong battle with depression felt: "You cannot think clearly about anything when you're depressed. You don't feel anything. It's like part of you left...The word depression has a real physical feeling – it feels like the world is pushing down, like there isn't any gravity, like you can't walk. It really is a state of body and mind."

According to the U.S. Center for Mental Health Services, up to half of all visits to doctors are depression-related, even if depression is never discussed. Problems such as chronic headaches, high blood pressure, fatigue, bowel problems and fibromyalgia can often be related to underlying depression.

By most estimates, depression – one of the most common forms of mental disorders – affects 20% of women, and it is two or three times higher in women than men. Some experts feel that statistic is true only because women are more willing to discuss and deal with their depression, while men may tend to mask it through workaholic tendencies, alcoholism or other kinds of behaviors.

Whatever the reason, depression is a real condition and it is treatable in a variety of ways. It can be caused by chemical imbalances and triggered by life changes, and people with a family history are at greater risk.

It's important to talk about it, not only with your doctor and health care team but with the people you must rely on for support – your family, friends, children, co-workers, etc.

Depression can be a dark, painful and lonely place, especially for women whose ideas about mental health are full of blame and shame.

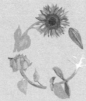 # TRIGGERS AND RISK FACTORS

Regardless of what causes an individual's depression, some life events are so powerful that they can trigger or worsen an existing problem. Common triggers include:

- Stressful job
- Children leaving home (the "empty nest" syndrome)
- History of previous depression or mental illness
- Family history of depression
- Unhappy or abusive marriage or relationship
- Financial problems and poverty
- Substance abuse (alcohol and other drugs)
- Certain medications
- Certain medical conditions (thyroid disorders, vitamin deficiencies, diabetes, chronic illness such as Parkinson's Disease, Alzheimer's Disease and Multiple Sclerosis)

MENTAL HEALTH & WELLNESS

Types of mental illness

According to Dr. Walter Smitson, Ph.D., Professor, Department of Psychiatry, University of Cincinnati Medical Center, President & CEO, Central Clinic, Inc., there are three major areas of mental illness: major depression, bipolar disorder and schizophrenia. Depression is, by far, the most common. Depression and related mental health problems are often difficult to diagnosis because they take several different forms. They include:

Clinical or major depression. Defined as any type of depression severe enough to require medical treatment, this type of depression can occur for a single definable period of time, such as a few weeks, or can linger for several months or more. It can occur more than once in a lifetime, too. Lingering depression is often called major depression or long-term depression.

Dysthymia. Recurrent or long-lasting depression, dysthymia (pronounced dis-THIGH-me-uh) is a mild form of depression or depressive thinking that may have existed for years or been present in a mild form since childhood or adolescence. People with dysthymia usually lack zest or enthusiasm and seem to drag through life, never fully satisfied or happy. Major depression and dysthymia are twice as common in women as in men.

Seasonal affective disorder. This is more common in northern climates and in winter months. It's a low or depressed feeling directly linked to lack of exposure to sunlight.

Postpartum depression. This type of depression affects new mothers, usually within a week to 6 months of delivery. It can interfere with the mother's ability to care for herself and her infant.

Panic disorder. Affecting twice as many women as men, panic disorders are irrational reactions to otherwise common events, characterized by rapid heart beat, feelings of impending doom, shortness of breath, sweaty palms and more. Some women mistake these symptoms for a heart attack. Be sure to check with your doctor if you have any of these symptoms.

Bipolar disorder. This is also treated as a form of depression, because depression is a serious part of this illness. Also called manic/depression, this up-down cycle is marked by tremendous mood swings – incredibly euphoric highs and very low lows.

Schizophrenia. Schizophrenia is a devastating brain disorder – the most chronic and disabling of the severe mental illnesses. The first signs of schizophrenia, which typically emerge in young people in their teens or twenties, are confusing and often shocking to families and friends. Hallucinations, delusions, disordered thinking, unusual speech and/or

Symptoms of Depression

According to the National Institutes of Mental Health (NIMH), depression should be considered if three or more of these symptoms persist more than two weeks or if they interfere with work or family life:

- Inappropriate crying spells.
- Persistent sad, anxious or "empty" moods and feelings.
- Loss of interest or pleasure in activities that used to bring pleasure – hobbies, sports, work, sex, art, music, etc.
- Feelings of guilt, worthlessness, hopelessness and pessimism.
- Sleeping too much or too little; awakening early in the morning.
- Eating too much or too little, with resulting weight gain or weight loss.
- Decreased energy levels, fatigue, a feeling of being "slowed down".
- Thoughts of death or suicide, or suicide attempts.
- Restlessness, irritability.
- Difficulty concentrating, remembering or making decisions.
- Persistent physical symptoms that do not respond to treatment, such as headaches, digestive disorders, chronic pain, dizziness, constipation, diarrhea, back pain, a "lump" in the throat, sexual dysfunction, abnormal heart rate, chest pain.

behavior and social withdrawal impair one's ability to interact with others. Most people with schizophrenia suffer chronically or episodically throughout their lives, losing opportunities for careers and relationships.

Moreover, people who suffer from depression tend to have worse health outcomes if they also have another disease – heart disease, cancer, diabetes, epilepsy or osteoporosis. Experts still don't know if the underlying disease worsens the depression or if the depression sets up the body for susceptibility to sickness.

A newsletter called *The Moody News*, written by and for people who struggle with depressive disorders, is a good window into what depression feels like and does to the people who experience it. Among their insights into depression and mental disorders, and beyond typical symptoms, this is how they say it affects everyday functioning:

Mental functions

You may have fewer ideas than normal or feel your thinking is slowed. You may be easily distracted, apathetic, bored, somber, afraid, stingy, envious or insecure. You may be oversensitive to criticism or feel frustrated when others challenge or oppose you.

Abnormal thinking

You may feel "down" on yourself, calling yourself ugly, sinful, guilty, worthless, unwanted, unloved or rejected by others. You may be over-anxious about your health, or worried about dying. You may have a foreboding sense of failure, incompetence, poverty or physical and mental defects.

Interactions with others

Your interactions with others may be affected. You may avoid others, act shy or aloof, try to avoid being noticed, assume blame, complain a lot or act submissive or passive to others. You may not be interested in relationships with others, avoiding interpersonal communication or becoming indifferent or hostile to others. Sex may not be interesting or important.

Actions and behaviors

You may procrastinate, be indecisive, cautious, obedient, inhibited, or resistant to change. Your speech or movement may become slow and quiet. People who are bipolar may become overly excited, impulsive, irritable, unable to sleep or have exaggerated beliefs in their abilities or powers.

Physical appearance

You may look older than your age, haggard, unkept or lack expression altogether. You may not care about your appearance or wardrobe, not caring about what you wear and not worried about your hair, skin, makeup or looks.

CAUSES

According to NIMH, several factors are at work in the development of depression. Experts aren't sure if it's a cause-effect relationship – whether certain factors, chemical imbalances or incidents cause depression, or whether those same factors evolve or worsen because of underlying depression.

The key factors related to depression are:

Genetic factors: Depression is more common in families with a history of depression, but that doesn't mean everyone in the family will experience it. Biochemistry, environmental stresses and other psychological or social factors play a role, too.

Biochemical factors: Brain chemistry that's out of balance is known to be a "significant factor" in depressive illnesses, the NIMH says. Most imbalances are related to brain chemicals called neurotransmitters, which regulate the messages delivered in the brain, to nerves and different parts of the body.

Environmental or other stresses: Life's events that represent major changes often trigger depression. These include significant loss, such as death or divorce, as well as difficult relationships, being a victim of sexual abuse or violence, financial problems or other major life changes. Sometimes, depression follows the onset of a chronic illness or open-heart surgery. Drug or alcohol abuse occurs in about one-third of people with depressive illnesses.

Psychological and social factors: People with certain temperaments or thought patterns seem to experience more depression. These might include people who are chronic pessimists, have low self-esteem, worry excessively or feel they have little control over situations.

TREATMENTS

Antidepressants. Most prescription drugs used to treat depression work by interacting with the brain chemicals that are linked to the disease. Usually they must be taken daily for at least 4 weeks or longer before people start noticing a difference (or decide to switch to another drug, if the first ones used do not work). For bipolar disorder, lithium is the treatment of choice because it helps even out mood swings. As with all drugs, discuss possible side effects, interactions, intended results and possible alternatives with your doctor and pharmacist.

Psychotherapy. Talking to a psychologist, psychiatrist or trained counselor can often be effective in overcoming depression, especially if combined with antidepressant drugs for severe cases. Mild to moderate cases of depression sometimes respond very well to therapy, according to NIMH, because people learn how to develop new behaviors, relationships or new ways of thinking about their disease and their interactions/reactions in the world.

Light therapy. For people suffering from Seasonal Affective Disorder, special light boxes can be placed around the house or at work to create the necessary spectrum of light needed to balance out the brain chemicals that get out of whack on long, dark days. Interior designers can also recommend changes to lighten the mood, brightness and appearance of rooms to help create a brighter, more supportive environment.

Herbal remedies. Several herbs are thought to be helpful for treating mild depression, including St. John's wort, ginkgo biloba and kava kava, although any treatment should be discussed with your doctor or pharmacist because of potential side effects or interactions with other drugs or conditions you may have.

Alternative treatments. Dr. Andrew Weil, author and director of integrative medicine at the University of Arizona, recommends several approaches for depression or anxiety disorders, including aerobic exercise, breath work (the deep breathing techniques used in yoga, for example) and meditation to calm the mind.

Exercise. Free to all who are willing to try, exercise is known to have tremendous benefits in fighting depression, because it counteracts the chemical imbalances in the body by producing feel-good endorphins and other brain chemicals that regulate mood. Exercise also has other benefits as well, including better heart health, better sleep patterns and better circulation. (See Chapter 2)

Dietary treatments. There is ongoing research into the potential benefits of Omega-3 fatty acids, found in salmon and sardines, fortified eggs, walnuts, soy, flax and hemp seeds (or in over-the-counter supplements), for combating bipolar disorder and depression.

Social support. Sometimes, treatment methods can be combined with support – formal or informal. Some people find that joining a support group helps them overcome feelings of isolation and also provides insights into how other people cope with similar problems.

If Others are Depressed

What if someone you love – a spouse, child or family member – struggles with depression?

- Don't blame the person for his/her feelings.
- Don't blame yourself for someone else's depression. Your responsibility is as a helper or facilitator, not someone who should or can take charge of someone else's mental health.
- Encourage the person to get screened or into treatment for depression or other mental disorders. Be supportive without being overbearing.
- Educate yourself and be a resource for someone else.

CHAPTER 14

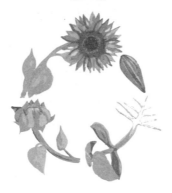

CANCER

Such great strides have been made in recent years regarding the detection and treatment of cancer, that what we now know for sure, is that a cancer diagnosis need no longer be a death sentence. Our knowledge, on the other hand, MUST be life-altering. Why? Prevention and early detection are key to boosting survival rates for almost any type of cancer.

Every woman's experiences with cancer are different, depending on her own encounters with the disease or the encounters of others in her life.

By their very makeup and the lifelong shifts of hormones, women may be prone to developing a variety of cancers throughout life, from skin cancers that develop as a result of sun worshipping to silent cancers of the ovaries to the very common breast cancers.

And no matter what your initial reaction, it's important to remember these facts:

⊛ Cancer is not a death sentence.

⊛ Many cancers can be prevented, and the decisions you make today and for the rest of your life can give you an edge in fighting cancer and reducing your risks. You greatly decrease your chances of developing cancer by altering your lifestyle, habits, diet and activity levels.

⊛ Many cancers, even the most serious, are treatable with a variety of approaches. Regardless of outcome, living with and surviving cancer are much easier today because of advances in treatment. The introduction of a variety of products and services, support networks and supportive therapies can help us deal with the disease and its effects. These include hair loss, fatigue, appetite loss, side effects from medicines or radiation, depression and fear.

⊛ According to the National Cancer Institute, up to 100,000 cancer deaths a year could be prevented by three measures – more exercise, a better diet that includes more whole grains and vegetables, and quitting smoking.

In this chapter, we'll look at some of the common cancers that affect women – what they are, how to reduce your risks, how they're treated and specific facts to know about each kind.

As with all serious diseases, having a sound medical team, in whom you trust, is a critical part of your treatment and recovery plan. Educating yourself is just as important as taking care of yourself throughout the entire cancer process.

PREVENTION

Cancer is a very simple disease. Actually, it means that abnormal cells develop and begin to grow, sometimes rapidly and sometimes slowly. But they cause abnormal clumps of cells, called tumors. Some tumors contain cells that are benign, meaning they're not cancerous and do not spread beyond the tumor itself. Some tumor cells are malignant, meaning they are cancerous and can spread to nearby tissue and other parts of the body. Once cancerous cells start to spread, usually through the blood system or lymphatic system, doctors call the tumor metastatic. (Metastasis is a word that means a "change," "passing over" or "transition.")

According to the American Cancer Society (ACS), all cancers caused by cigarette smoking and alcohol use could be prevented simply by not smoking and drinking only

155

moderately. And of the more than half million cancer-related deaths that occur each year in the U.S., nearly one-third are directly attributable to these factors:

* Obesity
* Poor nutrition
* Lack of exercise
* Other lifestyle factors, such as tobacco use, sun exposure, the use of certain medications or the existence of underlying disease

And many of those factors are controllable by lifestyle choices:

* Quit smoking
* Actively work to lose weight and keep it off
* Change from a diet of heavy, fatty, salty foods to those that are lower in fat and rich in fresh fruits and vegetables (at least 5 servings a day...a serving is only 1/2 cup)

The ACS points out that about half of all cancers can be detected by screening. So, getting regular checkups that include cancer screenings may reduce your risk and improve your chances of surviving cancer because treatment can start earlier, when it's more effective and successful.

The good news is that 62% of all people diagnosed with cancer survive at least 5 years, on average. Remember that this number includes people who were not detected early and whose cancer may have been quite advanced by the time they saw a doctor. Some survival rates are as high as 90% for some cancers, yet lower for others.

CANCER is a Gender-Specific Disease
The most common cancers in women are:

* Breast
* Ovarian
* Lung/bronchus
* Melanoma (skin cancer)
* Colon/rectum
* Non-Hodgkin's lymphoma
* Uterine

However, the cancers most likely to cause deaths in women, in order, are lung/bronchus, breast, colorectal, pancreas and ovarian.

BREAST CANCER

Ask any group of women, and a majority of them will identify breast cancer as their most pronounced health fear. Maybe it's because they know other women who've been treated for breast cancer. Maybe it's because the "one in eight women will get breast cancer in their lifetime" statistic has hit home more than once.

Facts about breast cancer: Except for non-melanoma skin cancers, breast cancer is the most frequently diagnosed cancer in women. Only lung cancer is more deadly than breast cancer.

Symptoms: Early breast cancer usually does not cause pain. In fact, when breast cancer first develops, there may be no symptoms at all. But as the cancer grows, it can cause changes that women should watch for:

⊛ A lump or thickening in or near the breast or in the underarm area.

⊛ A change in the size or shape of the breast.

⊛ A discharge from the nipple.

⊛ A change in the color or feel of the skin of the breast, areola or nipple (dimpled, puckered or scaly).

A woman should see her doctor if she notices any of these changes. Most often, they are not cancer, but only a doctor can tell for sure.

Who's at risk: The strange thing about breast cancer is that certain risk factors are associated with it, but many women with no risk factors and no history develop it. Still, it pays to know what's what. Common risk factors:

⊛ The older you are, the greater your risk of breast cancer.

⊛ If you got your period early in life or experienced a late menopause, you're at higher risk because your body has a longer lifetime exposure to estrogen.

⊛ Women who have never been pregnant seem to be at higher risk.

157

CANCER

- A family history of breast cancer (mother or sister) raises a woman's risk of breast cancer (although 85% of cancers are diagnosed in women with no family history), as does a family history of ovarian, endometrial or colon cancer (and prostate cancer in the men in your family).

- Women who use oral contraceptives or who take estrogen replacement therapy for menopause may be at increased risk.

- High-fat, low-fiber diet or excessive alcohol consumption may increase risk.

- Extensive radiation exposure and some environmental toxins/chemicals can increase risk.

- Researchers also have identified several genes that are markers for certain cancers, and women with those genes are at higher risk.

Early detection: The best ways to detect breast cancer is to combine monthly breast self-exams (See Chapter 6), yearly clinical exams by a health care provider and regular mammograms, especially after age 40, when the risk of breast cancer rises. Breast self-exams are good ways to spot changes in breast tissue over time, and mammograms can detect tiny cancers before physical symptoms develop.

Treatment: Treating breast cancer includes a variety of treatments: surgical removal of the tumor only or of the entire breast, chemotherapy, radiation, removal of surrounding lymph nodes, hormone therapy, or combinations of one or more treatments.

Consider the philosophy of empowering women to partner with their doctor about their health choices. "It's more complicated because we do have so many more choices for women now," says Rebecca Bechhold, M.D., a cancer specialist in Cincinnati. "When women come in for the first time with cancer, it's not a matter of saying, 'Let's do this,' " she explains, noting that each woman's cancer, health status and risk factors are different. " Instead, their doctor might say, 'Well, we can do this, or we can do something else, or given your age, we have these choices, too.' It really helps for women to be educated about what their choices are and about the various risks and benefits, because those are choices she'll have to make with her doctor."

Many women also feel pressed to make decisions quickly, Bechhold says. But she reassures women that there's always time to make a thoughtful, educated decision.

"It rarely is a rush decision, so women should feel free to take some time to really hash everything out with their doctor so they feel comfortable with their joint decisions."

Once breast cancer is treated, doctors also might recommend drugs – tamoxifen or anastrozole, for example – to reduce the possibility of its return. In truly severe cases – in women where cancer returns frequently or in families with extremely high rates of breast cancer in women – doctors sometimes recommend "preventive mastectomy," or removal of the breasts before cancer strikes. This is done to avoid the risk altogether, but is a severe decision that must be discussed in depth with your doctor, family, spouse and others.

Prevention: As with other cancers, regular exercise, maintaining a normal and healthy weight, reducing alcohol and eliminating tobacco are important in preventing cancer. Women are also urged to choose low-fat diets – less than 20% of a day's calories from fat – because as the breast ages, it harbors more fatty tissue than the breasts of younger women.

We're looking to men for help! Breast cancer is not exclusively a disease of women. For every 100 women with breast cancer, one male will develop the disease. The American Cancer Society estimates that 1,500 men will develop the disease this year. Moreover, many physicians and researchers believe that the answers to many questions regarding breast cancer may be found in the genetic makeup of men with the disease.

SKIN CANCER

It wasn't all that long ago when a deep, bronzed tan was the desired goal of summer, a time when no one had ever heard of sunscreens or SPF factors in creams, lotions and cosmetics.

CANCER

That's only one of the reasons that skin cancer – although not as deadly as others – is the most common cancer in the U.S. There are three types of skin cancer. **Squamous** cell cancer affects the outer layer of cells, **basal** cell cancer is in the layer of cells below the squamous cells, and **melanoma** (the most serious) affects cells in the deepest layers of the epidermis.

Facts: The numbers tell the story with skin cancer. More than a million cases of skin cancer are diagnosed each year, although only about 54,000 of them are melanomas, the most serious kind. Skin cancer is 10 times more common in whites that non-whites, but even individuals with dark, pigmented skin can develop skin cancer. One of the most common causes of skin cancer is exposure to the damaging ultra-violet radiation in sunlight. The sun's penetrating rays can damage the underlying structure and DNA in the skin. Equally (if not more) damaging is exposure to tanning beds, which provide intense ultraviolet rays to the skin.

Symptoms:

* Any change on the skin, especially in the size or color of a mole, growth or spot
* Scaly skin, oozing, bleeding or change in a bump or nodule
* Spread of pigmentation beyond the border of a mole or spot
* Change in sensation, itchiness, tenderness or pain

The American Cancer Society recommends the ABCD approach to checking your skin.

* **A** means "asymmetry," meaning one half of a mole does not match the other half.

* **B** means "border irregularity," in which the edges of a mole or spot are ragged, notched or blurred.

* **C** is for "color," because when cancerous skin changes color, it can take on several hues, including degrees of tan, brown, black, even streaks of dark blue and red.

* **D** is for "diameter," and any mole greater than 6 millimeters (about the size of a pencil eraser) should be checked.

Early Detection: Skin cancers are usually noticed because something changes – a mole, a spot, texture or color of the skin – so it's important to know what's normal.

Common Skin Cancer Sites

Examine your own skin regularly, and make sure your doctor checks the places you can't see (your back, the backs of your legs, the back of your neck/head) during your checkups.

15-20% of skin cancers occur here

25-30% here

35-40% here

Who's at risk: Anyone who spends a lot of time in the sun is at risk, and experiencing several scorching sunburns as a teenager seems to increase a person's risk of skin cancer as an adult. Others are at risk if they expose their skin to the lights in tanning beds, have a fair complexion, have lots of atypical moles or work in jobs where they're exposed to coal tar, pitch, creosote, arsenic compounds or radium.

Treatment: Almost all treatments for skin cancer include surgical removal of some kind. Some moles and cancers can be removed by burning, freezing or radiating them. Most of them are removed by traditional surgery, and doctors might also remove nearby lymph nodes to make sure the cancer hasn't spread. With severe cases, treatment might also include chemotherapy drugs and radiation.

Prevention: If you can, limit the amount of time you spend in the sun, especially between the hours of 10 a.m.-3 p.m. when the sun's rays are strongest. Wear hats and long sleeves when outdoors, and use a sunscreen with a sun protection factor of at least 15. The numbers in SPFs represent factors that indicate how much longer you can stay outside before burning. If you normally burn after 10 minutes, for example, using an SPF 15 lotion means you can stay out 15 times as long, or 150 minutes, before burning – but remember that sunscreens can wash off or wear off if you sweat or are active outside, so reapply often.

Did you know that an estimated 80% of a person's sun damage occurs before the age of 18? Research indicates that regular use of sunblock, with an SPF (Sun Protection Factor) of 15 or higher, during the first 18 years of life can lower the risk of certain skin cancers by 78%.

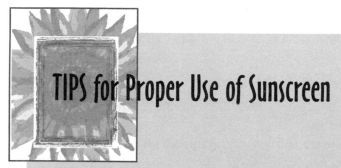

TIPS for Proper Use of Sunscreen

⊛ Apply sunscreen approximately 30 minutes before going outside, so that a good layer of protection can form.

⊛ Don't forget to apply sunscreen to your lips, hands, ears and feet.

⊛ Apply sunscreen generously to all areas of the body. Reapply approximately every 2 hours and after sweating or being in the water. Consider waterproof sunscreen.

⊛ Use protective eyewear (sunglasses, even for children) to shield eyes from the sun's harmful rays. Make certain the eyewear you choose provides 100% UV protection.

⊛ If taking prescription medication, consult your pharmacist to see if it may increase sensitivity to the sun.

⊛ Seek shade whenever possible – shaded structures such as trees and umbrellas provide great protection from the sun. Although trees do not offer complete sun protection, they do provide about 60 percent blockage from the sun's rays.

LUNG CANCER

Facts: The simple reality about lung cancer is that it probably wouldn't be such a common cancer if people didn't smoke tobacco. Nearly 80%-90% of all cancers are caused by smoking, and the risks are greater for people who have smoked more than 20 cigarettes a day since adulthood. Of all the cancers, it is the most preventable because it is most intimately linked with a lifestyle choice and habit. For women, it's not the cancer with the highest incidence, but it is the cancer that kills more women than any other – 68,000 or more a year.

Symptoms:

⊛ New, persistent cough or a change in a chronic cough

⊛ Chest pain, possibly a dull ache or sharp pain that's worse when inhaling

⊛ Shortness of breath, difficulty breathing

⊛ Wheezing

⊛ Abnormal curvature of the fingernails

Early Detection: There really is no way to detect lung cancer early, because it usually shows up on an X-ray of the lung after it already has developed.

Who's at Risk: Cigarette smoking is the leading risk factor for lung cancer – both for individuals who smoke and for non-smokers who breathe in second-hand smoke. Air pollution and tuberculosis are also possible risk factors for lung cancer, as are occupations that expose people to arsenic, some organic chemicals, radon, asbestos and radiation.

Treatment: Lung cancer is difficult to treat because it usually has spread to other parts of the body by the time it's diagnosed. Because of that, only about 15% of lung cancer patients survive up to five years. Doctors treat lung cancer with a variety of approaches, depending on the type of cancer, how far it has progressed and the health of the individual, but options include surgery, radiation and chemotherapy, or a combination of all three.

Prevention: Here, the advice is simple and straightforward: quit smoking! Even if you've smoked all your life, the minute you

CANCER

quit, you begin improving the health of your lungs (and heart and other organs) and reduce your risk of ever developing a respiratory disease. (See Chapter 12) Protect yourself and your family from second-hand smoke. Limit your exposure to cigarette smoking. Do not allow others to smoke in your home, avoid public places where smokers congregate, and encourage a smoke-free work environment. Be sure your child's care providers do the same.

CERVICAL CANCER

Facts: The introduction of the Pap smear as a screening test for cervical cancer has greatly reduced its incidence, but nearly 12,200 cases are diagnosed each year, with nearly twice as many cases in African-American women. In many women, there are no symptoms of cervical cancer. Their first indication of a problem is an abnormal Pap smear test result.

Symptoms:
- Abnormal vaginal or menstrual bleeding
- Bleeding after menopause
- Increased vaginal discharge

Early Detection: By age 18 or as soon as they become sexually active, all women should have a yearly Pap smear, which samples cells from the cervix for signs of abnormal or pre-cancerous changes. If a woman has a normal Pap test for several years in a row, her doctor may recommend a Pap smear every 2-3 years, although those who are in certain risk categories should be screened every year.

Who's at Risk: Women who have been sexually active with numerous partners are at greater risk of cervical cancer, especially if they're exposed to HPV, or human papilloma virus, an infection now directly linked to cervical cancer. Women who reach age 60 and have not had regular gynecological checkups or Pap smears are also more likely to develop cervical cancer. Others at high risk include women who began to have sex before age 16 or whose sexual partners may have had multiple partners. Smoking is also linked to cervical cancer.

Treatment: Doctors have several methods to treat cervical cancer, depending on how advanced it is. The cancerous cells can be removed by burning or freezing them, exposing them to laser treatment or removing them surgically. Radiation and chemotherapy, or both, also may be recommended for some types of cancers.

Prevention: Practicing safe sex, limiting the number of sexual partners and having regular gynecologic checkups from puberty through postmenopausal years, can help reduce the risk of cervical cancer. Some research suggests that diets high in Vitamin C (citrus fruits, broccoli, strawberries, chili peppers, papaya, cantaloupe) and Vitamin E (supplements) can reduce cervical cancer risks.

OVARIAN CANCER

Facts: Of all the cancers that affect a woman's reproductive system, none cause as many deaths (14,300 a year) as ovarian cancer, or cancer of the ovaries.

Symptoms:

- Enlargement of the abdomen (fluid accumulation)
- Stomach discomfort, gas, bloating
- Abnormal vaginal bleeding (rare)

Early Detection: Whenever a doctor performs a pelvic exam, it's usually to feel the ovaries inside the body and make sure that they have not become inflamed, swollen or surrounded by fluid. A CA125 test can diagnose ovarian cancer once it's suspected, but there really is no test to detect it beforehand.

Who's at Risk: As women get older, their risks for ovarian cancer increase. Also at risk are women who've never had children and those who have used fertility drugs or hormone replacement therapy. Being pregnant, having a tubal ligation (sterilization by severing the fallopian tubes) or using oral contraceptives actually appear to reduce the risk of ovarian cancer. Two unproven but possible risk factors, according to the ACS, include the use of talcum powder in the area between the vagina and anus, and eating a high-fat diet.

CANCER

Treatment: Sometimes, it is possible for a doctor to remove only the cancerous ovary, especially if the woman is young enough and still wants to have children. However, treatment often includes surgical removal of the ovaries and the uterus (hysterectomy), or a combination of surgery, radiation and chemotherapy.

Prevention: Make sure your regular checkup includes a pelvic exam, eat a diet low in fat, avoid the use of talcum powder on infants and on yourself in the genital area, and make informed choices throughout life about the use of certain medicines and drugs.

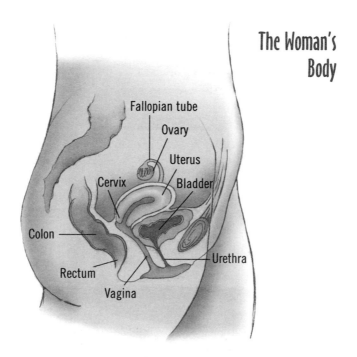

The Woman's Body

Fallopian tube

Ovary

Uterus

Cervix

Bladder

Colon

Rectum

Urethra

Vagina

ENDOMETRIAL CANCER

Another type of gynecological cancer is endometrial cancer. It develops in the lining of the uterus, or endometrium. Although it's more common in Caucasians than in African-American women, the mortality rates are higher in African-American women. If you experience abnormal vaginal bleeding or spotting after menopause, or abdominal/pelvic pain, ask your doctor to consider an endometrial screening – a test to examine the cells of the endometrium.

COLON CANCER

Facts: Colon cancer, also called colorectal cancer, is the third most common cancer in women (and men). Like several other cancers, it's often a "silent" disease because it may exist without symptoms. However, it is a very preventable cancer because early detection and removal of polyps in the colon and rectum can prevent the development of cancer.

Symptoms:

✿ Rectal bleeding, blood in the stool

✿ Change in bowel habits

✿ Cramping pain in the lower abdomen

Early Detection: The tests used to screen for colorectal cancer have strange-sounding names, such as sigmoidoscopy, colonoscopy, barium enema and fecal occult blood tests. Basically, they're all tests that either examine the insides of the colon and rectum to look for polyps – tissue growths in the colon – or to test for signs of blood in the stool. At age 50, women should have a fecal occult blood test annually (done at home by collecting a sample of stool and sending it to a lab for analysis), and a sigmoidoscopy every five years, with colonoscopy or barium enema recommended every 5-10 years, depending on risk. A digital rectal exam, usually performed during regular checkups or these tests, involves inserting a finger into the rectum to feel for normal tissue. Those with a family history of colon cancer may need to be tested earlier and more often. Some doctors believe that African Americans may be at higher risk for colon cancer, and should therefore be screened earlier and more often. Speak to your doctor about your risk factors.

Who's at Risk: The older you are, the greater your risk for colorectal cancer. Most cases occur after age 50, although other factors are involved. People with a family history of colorectal cancer, polyps or inflammatory bowel disease seem to have higher risks for colorectal cancer. A risk of ovarian, endometrial or breast cancer is also associated with a higher likelihood of developing colorectal cancer. High risk behaviors include: smoking, alcohol consumption, obesity, lack of exercise, a diet high in fat or low in fiber, inadequate intake of fruits and vegetables.

Treatment: Usually, doctors must remove all or part of the colon and/or rectum to treat colorectal cancer, and surgery is usually effective. If cancer has spread to nearby tissue or organs, chemotherapy and radiation might be recommended before or after surgery.

Prevention: First, tackle your diet by adding more fiber, fresh fruits and vegetables, especially leafy green vegetables, and cutting back on saturated fat, especially red meats and processed meat. If you smoke, quit. And consider taking an aspirin a day. Researchers have found that a daily aspirin may reduce the number and size of polyps – tiny tissue growths inside the colon that are benign but can sometimes turn into cancerous tumors.

Education and knowledge are your best allies in preventing or detecting cancers. Know your family history and lifestyle risk factors and communicate these to your doctor. Partnering with your doctor will help you make the right choices. Be sure to share this information with other members of your family, including the next generations.

CHAPTER 15

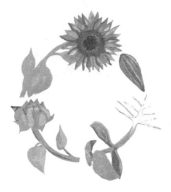

HOME FIRST AID

Women tend to take care of a lot of people in their lives – children, husbands, friends, neighbors, aging parents, even the kids next door, on occasion.

Most of their caretaking is an ongoing occurrence, but every once in a while, they're called on to care for someone immediately. Perhaps a child falls and breaks an arm, or a co-worker collapses in the throes of an asthma attack at work. Maybe it's a soccer game suddenly invaded by stinging honeybees or a car accident that finds them binding a bleeding wound or worse, dealing with a head, neck or spinal injury. Knowing what to do, and sometimes, more importantly, what "not" to do, may make the difference between life and death, permanent disability or possible recovery.

Women who know first aid are women who know how to help, and in today's world, "first aid" can mean everything from recognizing heart attack and stroke symptoms, to providing emergency wound care, to having the right supplies on hand in the family medicine cabinet.

HOME FIRST AID

Based on guidelines from the American Red Cross, this chapter will give you plenty of information on general medical care in the home and first aid anywhere. Because you never know when you might need it!

THE FAMILY MEDICINE CHEST

If you think ahead, many of the products, items and pieces of equipment you need to handle minor health problems and emergencies at home will be waiting for you when you need them. So next time you make a trip to the store or pharmacy, make a checklist and stock up on the necessary items for a well-equipped home medicine kit.

Among the things to keep on hand, according to Wal-Mart Pharmacist Karen Froendhoff:

- Adhesive tape and adhesive bandages of all sizes and shapes
- Alcohol wipes
- Antacids
- Antibacterial soap (or antibacterial hand sanitizer for times when you don't have access to water)
- Antibiotic ointment to prevent infection of cuts, wounds or abrasions
- Anti-diarrhea medicine
- Antihistamine to relieve allergy symptoms or allergy attacks, including soothing eye drops
- Cough syrup
- Decongestant to relieve coughs due to colds and flu
- Disposable gloves (to prevent contact with someone else's blood or body fluids)
- Disposable hot wrap and refreezable ice pack
- Elastic band or rubber hose to use as a tourniquet
- Fever-reducing medicine (such as acetaminophen)

WARNING: Do not give aspirin to children under 12. Ask your doctor or pharmacist for a substitute. Children given aspirin are at risk for a reaction called Reye's syndrome.

* Gauze pads
* Hydrocortisone cream to relieve itching and swelling
* Measuring spoon
* Mentholated chest rub for chest congestion
* Pain-relievers (ibuprofen, acetaminophen, aspirin – but do not give aspirin to children)
* Saline-solution eyewash
* Scissors
* Sinus medication to relieve pain and pressure
* Syrup of ipecac to induce vomiting if poisons have been ingested AND activated charcoal to absorb ingested poison. **WARNING: Use these products ONLY after talking with your doctor or receiving advice from a drug/poison information center.** In the event of accidental poisoning, it is essential that you have these items available for use upon the specific instruction of the poison control center or 911.
* Thermometer
* Tongue depressor or frozen-treat sticks to use for small splints
* Tweezers

Clearly, you won't use most of these items on a regular basis (or ever, if you're lucky!), but in case the need ever arises, it's nice to know that you're prepared.

How old is this stuff? Upkeep of the medicine cabinet

Every once in a while, it's a good idea to conduct "spring cleaning" in the medicine chest. Over-the-counter and prescription drugs can lose their effectiveness or turn stale over time. So keep these points in mind:

* Check expiration dates on medicines and throw away those that are outdated. If you're not sure, call your pharmacist and ask what the drug's shelf life is.
* Keep medicines in their original containers and labeled clearly. Throw out those that are not identified or no

longer necessary. (Flushing is a good way to get rid of them.)

⊛ Every medicine and product stored in a bathroom – vitamins, herbs, over-the-counter drugs, prescription drugs, cosmetics, cleaning products, etc. – is a potential poison. Keep them out of reach of children or locked in a high cabinet.

⊛ Many medicine labels say "store in a cool, dry place." If your medicine chest is in a hot, steamy bathroom, find another suitable storage place, such as a high shelf in a hallway linen closet or a kitchen cabinet.

⊛ Give medicines only to the family members for whom they were prescribed.

⊛ Always read directions and doses.

⊛ If you're taking or giving medicine at night, turn on the light so you're sure you have the right product.

FIRST AID BASICS

If the last time you learned basic first aid was in grade school or high school, much of the information has not changed, but much is new, too.

The rise in the spread of blood borne disease, including AIDS and hepatitis, has led to a whole new emphasis on protecting one's self from exposure to another person's blood or body fluids. Although the risk of contracting a disease is rare, according to the American Red Cross, the following precautions can reduce your risk:

1. Avoid contact with blood and other body fluids.

2. Use protective equipment, such as disposable gloves (available at any drug store) and breathing masks.

3. Thoroughly wash your hands with soap and water immediately after giving care to someone else.

If you do have to clean up a blood spill, do so immediately or as soon as possible after it occurs. Use disposable gloves and a breathing barrier, and wipe up the spill with paper towels or other absorbent material. Then flood the area with a solution of water and bleach (one gallon of water, 1/4 cup bleach), allow it to stand for 20 minutes and then wipe it carefully. Throw away all material used in the cleanup in a labeled biohazard container.

Treating shock: ABC's

No matter what the injury, someone administering first aid should always be on the lookout for shock. Shock means that the body has suffered a tremendous injury or trauma of some kind. Shock can be brought on by a severe injury, loss of blood, a life-threatening allergic reaction, poisoning or other event.

When shock occurs, the body's blood pressure drops suddenly, and the heart is not able to provide enough blood to the body's tissues. Signs of shock include:

- Restlessness or irritability
- Nausea and vomiting
- An altered level of consciousness (confused or dazed)
- Pale or ashen skin; cool or moist skin
- A blue tinge to the lips and fingernails
- Rapid or shallow breathing
- Rapid heartbeat

What to do if you suspect shock:

- Call 911
- Monitor the victim's ABC – airway, breathing and circulation
- Control any external bleeding
- Keep the victim from getting chilled or overheated
- Elevate the victim's legs about 12 inches – but only if you do not suspect a head, neck or back injury or do not suspect broken bones in the hips or legs

WARNING – IF THERE IS ANY CHANCE OF TRAUMA OR SEVERE INJURY TO THE HEAD, NECK OR SPINAL CORD, NEVER, EVER ATTEMPT TO MOVE THE VICTIM. MOVING THE VICTIM COULD FURTHER DAMAGE THE

SPINAL CORD CAUSING PERMANENT PARALYSIS OR BRAIN INJURY. THE ONLY EXCEPTION TO THIS RULE IS IF THE VICTIM IS UNDER WATER. IN THIS INSTANCE, BRING THE VICTIM TO THE SURFACE TO ENABLE BREATHING, TAKING CARE TO SUPPORT THE HEAD AND NECK AS MUCH AS POSSIBLE.

* Comfort and reassure the victim until advanced medical personnel arrive and take over. Do not give food or drink to someone in shock.

Controlling bleeding:
If someone is bleeding, follow these steps:

* Put on disposable gloves to protect yourself.

* Cover the wound with a dressing (gauze, clean cloth) and press firmly and directly against the wound.

* Elevate the injured area so that it is held above the victim's heart – but do this ONLY when you suspect that a bone is not broken.

* Cover the wound by rolling it in gauze or a dressing, tear small strips at the end and tie a knot directly over the wound.

* If the bleeding does not stop, apply additional dressing and bandages. Apply pressure directly to the wound to squeeze the artery against the bone and call 911 or have someone near you call 911. Look for signs of shock.

Special injury situations

Eye injuries: If someone injures the eye or has an object embedded in the eye, do not attempt to remove the object. Place the victim in a comfortable position and place a sterile dressing around the eye and the object, stabilizing it as best you can. Apply a bandage but do not put direct pressure on the eyeball. Seek medical treatment as soon as possible.

Chemicals in the eye: Quick treatment is required if chemicals or other dangerous substances get into the eye, because blindness or permanent damage can occur quickly. Symptoms of eye contamination include extreme pain, and the victim may or not be able to open the affected eye. Usually, the eye will water a lot, become red and swell. Suggestions for treatment include:

- Do not touch the victim's eye, and don't let the victim touch it, either. Put on protective gloves, if possible.
- Hold the victim's head under a water faucet so that water runs over the eye for at least 10 minutes. Make sure the water that rinses away from the eye does not splash you or the victim, because it can be contaminated, too. If a faucet is not available or does not accommodate someone's head underneath it, use a pitcher or glass to pour the water.
- If the victim cannot open the eye, gently pull apart the eyelids to clean all parts of the eye and eyelids.
- Place a sterile pad or clean pad made of non-fluff materials over the eye, and ask the victim to hold it in place. If possible, identify the chemical or substance that caused the problem, and make sure the victim is treated in an emergency room.

Nosebleed: Lean the victim **forward** (Yes, forward!) and pinch the nostrils together until bleeding stops.

Tooth knocked out: Place a sterile dressing directly in the space left by the tooth and ask the victim to bite down gently to apply direct pressure. Preserve the tooth by placing it in a container of cool, fresh milk or water. Always try to handle the tooth by the chewing edge, not the root. Get the victim and the tooth to a dentist immediately. The sooner the victim is treated, the better the chance of saving and re-implanting the tooth.

Preventing choking

Many people, and especially young children, can choke on even common objects.

First, make sure you do everything possible to prevent choking from happening. Put children in a high chair or at a table while they eat, and do not let them eat too fast. Give infants soft foods that don't require chewing. Supervise children while they eat, and cut food into small bites until

HOME FIRST AID

infants and children learn how to chew their food completely.

Dangerous foods that should not be given to children under the age of 4 include: hot dogs, nuts, chunks of meat or cheese, hard or sticky candy, popcorn, raw carrots, whole grapes, chunky peanut butter.

Dangerous household items that should be stored out of the reach of children and infants include: balloons, coins, marbles, small toy parts, pen or marker caps, small button-type batteries, small compressible toys that can fit entirely in a child's mouth and plastic bags. Do not, however, assume that this list is complete. When in doubt, take it away. If a child can possibly put it into the mouth, it will go into the mouth. Never leave a child unattended! Remember, your toddler can find things even your vacuum cleaner misses.

Treating choking: The Heimlich Maneuver

Lung specialist, Dr. Henry Heimlich, changed medical history when he educated the public about a maneuver to expel foreign objects that are stuck in the windpipes of choking individuals. Rather than slapping people on the back, Heimlich popularized a technique that uses air already inside the lung to expel the object out, not lodge it in further.

Today, the Heimlich Maneuver is a standard first-aid intervention for choking and drowning, and the Heimlich Institute also recommends it to treat asthma attacks as well.

A choking victim can't speak or breathe and needs your help immediately. **If possible, dial 911 as you begin the Heimlich Maneuver, or send someone for help while you work with the victim. Follow these steps to help a choking victim:**

1. From behind, wrap your arms around the victim's waist.

2. Make a fist and place the thumb side of your fist against the victim's upper abdomen, below the ribcage and above the navel.

176

3. Grasp your fist with your other hand and press into their upper abdomen with a quick upward thrust. Do not squeeze the ribcage. Confine the force of the thrust to your hands.

4. Repeat until the object is expelled.

If the victim is unconscious, or if you can't reach around the victim, place the victim on the back. Facing the victim, kneel astride the victim's hips. With one of your hands on top of the other, place the heel of your bottom hand on the upper abdomen below the rib cage and above the navel. Use your body weight to press into the victim's upper abdomen with a quick upward thrust. Repeat until the object is expelled. If the victim has not recovered, proceed with rescue breathing, or cardiopulmonary resuscitation.

Whatever you do when dealing with someone who is choking, do not slap the victim's back. Doing so can lodge the object even further into the windpipe.

Did you know it's also possible to perform the Heimlich Maneuver on yourself? Suppose you're at home alone and begin to choke on a piece of candy or chunk of meat. What would you do? Here's how to help yourself.

1. Make a fist and place the thumb side of your fist against your upper abdomen, below the ribcage and above the navel.

2. Grasp your fist with your other hand and press into your upper abdomen with a quick upward thrust.

3. Repeat until object is expelled.

If that does not work, you can also lean over a fixed horizontal object (table edge, chair, railing) and press your upper abdomen against the edge to produce a quick upward thrust. Repeat until the object is expelled.

After having choking first aid administered, the victim should see a physician immediately, according to the Heimlich Institute.

INFANT CHOKING

Few things are more frightening than the sight of an infant choking, and babies can choke very easily on common objects. According to the American Red Cross, a child who is coughing should be allowed to continue coughing in hopes of expelling the object. If the baby's face turns red, and then blue, or if a baby's cries become high-pitched, call 911 for help and intervene with anti-choking measures.

There are two schools of thought on how to treat an infant who is choking. Below, we've outlined both the **Heimlich Institute's** recommendation and the **American Red Cross** method. Familiarize yourself with both and discuss with your pediatrician which he or she recommends. This way, you'll be prepared to act in the event of an emergency.

The Red Cross recommends that you lay the infant face down on your forearm or lap, with the baby's head lower than the trunk. Support the baby's head and shoulders with your hand, grasping the jaw gently with your thumb and forefinger. Use the heel of your hand and give up to 5 sharp slaps – firm but without causing injury – between the infant's shoulders.

⊛ If back slaps are not effective, shift the infant to your other arm in a face-up position with the head lower than the body, supporting the back with your hand. Place two fingers on the lower half of the baby's breastbone. Give 5 sharp inward and downward thrusts into the chest. Continue with back slaps and chest thrusts until help arrives.

⊛ Never reach into a baby's throat to remove an object, because you might actually push it farther into the airway. Remove an object only if you can see it and can remove it without lodging it farther into the throat.

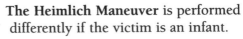

The Heimlich Maneuver is performed differently if the victim is an infant.

You can choose from one of two positions. Hold the sitting infant on your lap with the baby facing away from you. Reach around the infant and place your middle and index fingers of both your hands below the baby's ribcage and above the navel. You may also lay the child down, face up, on a firm surface and kneel or stand at the baby's feet. Place the middle and index fingers of both your hands below the baby's rib cage and above the navel (see drawing). Press into the baby's upper abdomen with a quick upward thrust; do not squeeze the rib cage. Be very gentle. Repeat until the object is expelled.

Sprains, strains and fractures

Injuries to different body parts require different actions.

Leg injury: Immobilize the injured leg by binding it (with gauze or strips of material) to the uninjured leg.

Foot injuries: Immobilize the ankle and foot using a soft splint, such as a pillow or rolled blanket. Do not remove the shoes.

Rib/breastbone fracture: Place a folded blanket or pillow between the injured ribs and the arm. Bind the arm to the body (with rolled gauze or strips of material) to help support the injured area.

Hand/finger injuries: Apply a bulky dressing to the injured area. If the finger looks fractured or is dislocated, tape the injured finger to the finger next to it. If possible, remove any jewelry from the injured area as soon as possible.

Injured? Think R.I.C.E.!

R.I.C.E. stands for Rest, Ice, Compression and Elevation. It may help control pain and swelling and minimize the side effects of an injury. Severe or persistent pain or swelling may require immediate medical attention.

HOME FIRST AID

BRRRRrrrrrr...It's cold

Being exposed to the cold for too long can bring on hypothermia or frostbite, both of which require first-aid treatment.

When someone develops hypothermia, they will shiver, become apathetic, develop impaired judgment, have a slow and irregular pulse, experience numbness and have a glassy stare.

- Gently move the victim to a warm place, if possible.
- Check ABCs (airway, breathing, circulation) and care for shock.
- Remove wet clothing and cover the victim with blankets or plastic sheeting to keep in body heat.
- Warm the victim slowly and handle the victim carefully.

Frostbite...Even colder

When exposed to extremely cold temperatures, individual cells can freeze and begin to die. That's frostbite.

Symptoms of frostbite include: loss of feeling and sensation, especially in the extremities (fingers, toes, tip of the nose, ears); skin that's discolored and waxy-looking; blisters and blue skin in severe cases.

How to treat frostbite: Remove wet clothing and jewelry from the affected area and soak the frostbitten area(s) in warm (not hot) water. Cover with dry, sterile dressings but do not rub frostbitten tissue. Check ABCs and care for shock. Seek medical help.

Boy...It's hot!

Heat, sun and humidity take their toll on the body, too. When the body overheats, the body begins to shut down to preserve critical inner organs and tissues. The American Red Cross defines three basics types of heat-related conditions:

Heat cramps are characterized by painful muscle spasms, usually in the legs and abdomen. Move the victim to a cool place and offer cool water to drink. Ask the victim to stretch the muscle lightly, and gently massage the area.

Heat exhaustion is characterized by skin that turns cool and moist and looks flushed, pale or ashen. Other symptoms include headache, dizziness, nausea, weakness and exhaustion. Move the victim to a cooler environment and loosen or remove clothing. Fan the victim to create circulating air while you apply water with a cloth or sponge. If the victim is conscious, give small sips of cool water to drink, and if the symptoms do not improve, call 911.

Heat stroke is the most serious of all heat-related emergencies. Victims will experience a change in the level of consciousness, have a high body temperature, rapid or weak pulse and rapid or shallow breathing. Skin may look red and feel hot and can be either dry or moist. Call 911 immediately and provide the same care as suggested for heat exhaustion until help arrives.

CPR – cardiopulmonary resuscitation
CPR is a form of intervention, usually administered to someone whose heart has stopped beating and who is no longer breathing. If only the breathing has stopped, rescue breathing alone can be administered to keep air flowing in and out of the lungs.

CPR is a two-stage approach in which the person providing first aid keeps pumping the victim's heart to keep blood flowing and blows air into the lungs to keep oxygen circulating through the body. It's always done until professional emergency medical help arrives.

FIRST, CALL 911 FOR EMERGENCY HELP.
To administer CPR:
First, lay the victim on his/her back. Find the correct position for your hands on the victim's chest. Using your hand that's closest to the victim's feet, use two fingers to locate the notch on the lower end of the victim's sternum (the breastbone, or bottom of the rib cage). Slide your middle and index fingers up to the edge of the rib cage to that notch where the ribs meet the breastbone. Place your middle finger in the notch, your index finger above it, and the heel of your other hand just above your index finger on the breastbone. This is the area of the chest

where you must apply downward pressure. Now place the heel of your first hand on top of the other hand, interlocking the fingers so that the fingers of bottom hand are raised off the victim's chest.

1. Give 15 compressions, or downward thrusts. Position your shoulders over your hands and compress the chest – pushing downward – about two inches. Do 15 compressions in about 10 seconds, and keep the up-and-down movements smooth. Keep your hand in contact with the victim's chest at all times.

2. Now shift to the person's head and mouth to give rescue breaths. Open the person's airway by tilting the head backwards and lifting the chin. Pinch the victim's nose shut and seal your lips tightly around the person's mouth. Give two rescue breaths into the person's mouth, each lasting about 2 seconds. Watch the victim's chest rise to be sure your breaths go in.

3. Repeat the compression/breathing cycles – 3 more sets of 15 compressions and 2 more breathing rescue sessions.

4. After one minute, check the person's circulation for no more than 10 seconds…look, listen and feel for breathing.

5. If the person has a pulse and is breathing, keep the airway open, monitor the breathing and wait for emergency help to arrive.

6. If the person has a pulse but still is not breathing, continue to do rescue breathing and check the circulation signs about every minute. Wait for medical help to arrive.

7. If the person has no pulse and is not breathing, continue administering CPR – 15 compressions followed by 2 rescue breaths – until help arrives, checking the person's pulse every few minutes.

Why is it important to perform rescue breathing?

When the body is deprived of oxygen, the brain begins to die within 4-6 minutes. Rescue breathing is a way of keeping oxygen flowing into the person's lungs and throughout the bloodstream if the victim is unconscious or is having a breathing emergency – an asthma attack, for example, or is in shock. And when it comes to rescue breathing, time is of the essence.

MINUTES COUNT, AND BRAIN DAMAGE CAN OCCUR QUICKLY

⊛ In the first minute of not breathing: the heart will soon stop beating, too.

⊛ 4-6 minutes without breathing: brain damage is possible.

⊛ 6-10 minutes without breathing: brain damage is likely.

⊛ 10 or more minutes without breathing: irreversible brain damage is certain.

Be Prepared...

The most important item to have in a medical emergency is information. Doctors suggest that you keep a written record of each family member's medical history. In the event of an emergency, when your emotions are at their peak, the health care professionals need information that may save your loved one's life. Include:

⊛ *Allergies. List any medication, food or latex allergies or sensitivities your family member may have or has had.*

⊛ *An updated list of your family's medications, including dosage.*

⊛ *Any pre-existing illness or surgeries. Don't leave anything out.*

If a family member has a chronic condition such as diabetes or asthma, or is allergic to medications, doctors suggest that they wear an identifying alert bracelet or necklace. In an emergency, this could save your loved one's life. In the event of an asthma attack, the victim should not be left alone until the attack has subsided with proper use of inhaled medications. If the inhaler is not readily available, accompany the victim to the location of the inhaler. Each moment is precious.

Home Safety Tips

* Apply sunscreen approximately 30 minutes before going outside, so that a good layer of protection can form.

* Be certain your home is equipped with smoke and fire detectors, as well as a fire extinguisher in the kitchen, garage, workshop or other areas where fire may occur. Check batteries in each detector twice a year.

* Be certain your home is free of carbon monoxide gases. At-home detectors are available.

* Teach your children what to do in the event of a fire in the home. Have a fire drill. Be sure second-floor bedrooms have more than one escape route. Consider a collapsible ladder for upper floor bedrooms.

* You should check your first-aid kit once a year – maybe the same day you check your smoke and carbon monoxide detectors – to make sure it is well stocked and no medications have expired.

* If you have children in your home, take care to childproof it. This includes safety latches on cabinets and doors, closed doors near stairways, child-proof caps on medications, locked poisons and household detergents and child safety barriers in electrical outlets.

* If you keep guns or firearms in the house, be sure they are stored in a locked cabinet. Consider storing bullets in a separate locked location. Talk to your older children about gun safety.

* Teach your children to practice safe habits around strange animals, even if they belong to a neighbor. Animals can be unpredictable. Always ask for permission from the owner before allowing your child to approach an animal.

* Learn CPR!!!! (See pages 181-183)

* Learn what to do if your child or someone is choking. (See pages 176-179)

* Require regular babysitters to take a basic first-aid class. The American Red Cross offers classes to young babysitters.

* **Teach your child to call 911 in the event of an emergency. Even very young children can save lives.**

Index

Index